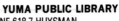

D0427457

A MOTHER'S TEARS

UNDERSTANDING
THE MOOD SWINGS
THAT FOLLOW
CHILDBIRTH

Arlene M. Huysman, Ph.D.
Foreword by Paul J. Goodnick, M.D.

SEVEN STORIES PRESS / New York

In the U.K.: Turnaround Publisher Services Ltd., Unit 3, Olympia Trading Estate,
Coburg Road, Wood Green, London N22 6TZ, U.K.

In Canada: Hushion House, 36 Northline Road, Toronto, Ontario M4B 3E2, Canada

Library of Congress Cataloging-in-Publication Data
Huysman, Arlene.
    A Mother's Tears: Understanding the Mood Swings that Follow Childbirth/
    Arlene Huysman.
        p. cm.
    ISBN 1-888363-70-3 (cloth)
    1. Postpartum depression I. Title
RG852.H89 1998
618.7'6—dc21   97-52079
                                                 CIP

Book design by Cindy LaBreacht

Seven Stories Press
140 Watts Street
New York, NY 10013

Printed in the U.S.A.

10 9 8 7 6 5 4 3 2 1

To my dear husband, Pedro,
my wonderful children, Pam and Jamie,
their spouses, Steve and Betsy,

and
the very special Andrea Maxine

CONTENTS

ACKNOWLEDGMENTS

MANY PEOPLE come to mind as I recall how difficult it was to make the decision to write this book. I knew that the subject would generate controversy and conflicting opinions. This book is not intended to be scientifically definitive. Rather it is written to address the myths surrounding the postpartum period in a woman's life and the perspectives of the legal and medical communities. My theories are born out of my many years of professional experience and from the knowledge I have gained as a clinical psychologist from my patients and colleagues.

Therefore it is important to acknowledge all who preceded me in the attempt to bring attention to the sufferings of new mothers. I have heavily relied on the work of writers and researchers in the field of postpartum, depression, and manic-depression. These include Carol Dix, author of *The New Mother Syndrome;* Dr. James Alexander Hamilton and Patricia Neel Harberger, M.S., editors of *Postpartum Psychiatric Illness: A Picture Puzzle;* Dr. Carl S. Burak and Michele G. Remington, authors of *The Cradle Will Fall;* Dr. Mark S.

Gold, author of *The Good News About Depression;* Drs. Kay Redfield Jamison and Frederick K. Goodwin for their book *Manic-Depressive Illness,* a bible of diagnosis and treatment; and Dr. Jamison for her book *The Unquiet Mind;* Deanne Tilton Durfee for her involvement in "A Nation's Shame: Fatal Child Abuse and Neglect in the United States"; Drs. Steven J. Shea and Geoffrey R. McKee, researchers and forensic experts; Patty Duke and Gloria Hochman for *A Brilliant Madness;* and Ronald R. Fieve, M.D., for *Moodswing.* These works provided me a starting place for my own research and theory. In many cases I have quoted these professionals, sometimes to add my voice of agreement, and sometimes to disagree, but in all instances, to emphasize the importance of their writings.

I am grateful for my associations with so many fine clinicians: psychiatrists, psychologists, social workers, nurses, marriage and family counselors, and clergy with whom I had the privilege to practice and share cases and who, in turn, shared their cases with me. These included Arnold L. Lieber, M.D, who reviewed my manuscript meticulously; Warren Schlanger, M.D; the late Fransciso Bolea, M.D, my friend and former associate; Paul Goodnick, M.D, researcher and author; Jan Maizler, LCSW, my associate for many years; Lavanne Warren, ARNP; Joan Levi, LCSW; Victoria Haefner, LCSW; Elona Kurosad, R.N., friend and associate; Paul Inkeles, Ph.D.; my courageous sister, Bernice Diamond; Rabbi Eugene Labovitz, friend and spiritual advisor; the many interns, especially Irene Bravo, who read and commented on my work; and with me always in spirit are my mother and father, Anna and Max Weiss.

I wish to add a special note in acknowledgment of the late Gaston Magrinat, M.D., my first mentor. He taught me, along with countless others, the ability to recognize and treat manic-depression. He shared with us his knowledge and understanding of scientific tests, measurements, interview techniques, and lithium carbonate treatment, as well as an understanding of the essence of the disease and those who are prone to suffer from it. His contribution has proliferated through an ever increasing professional circle, saving multitudes of patients.

My wonderful and patient husband, Pedro Camacho, assumed many of my responsibilities so that I could devote myself to this book. I am forever grateful to him for sharing his quiet faith in my abilities. My sensitive and gifted children, Pam Koretsky and James Huysman—both excellent clinicians in their own right—cheered me on, contributed research and opinions, and buoyed me up when my energies flagged.

Both for support at home and at work I thank Judy Schlanger, my long-time right hand; Cele Wallach; Marta Santiago; Bonnie Rionda; and all those made it possible to complete the project.

Those most closely associated with the writing of this book are: Laura Brown, who helped me inaugurate this project, and Shelby Brown, my agent, who believed in the project and who did not give up until she found a publisher who understood its necessity in educating expectant mothers and their families. The publisher and editor, Dan Simon of Seven Stories Press, quickly recognized what I intended this book to be. His advice was vital. Thanks also to Mikola De Roo for her patience and diligent, cogent editing. And last but not least, Laura Cerwinske, author, writing teacher, and philosopher, was always readily available to help organize both my thoughts and the manuscript, for which I am eternally grateful. She has enriched my life enormously.

FOREWORD

PUBLICATION OF this book on mood swings after childbirth highlights an area of growing focus, i.e., those mood changes that occur specifically in the female gender. For too long, it has been assumed that depression in both sexes is exactly the same, despite the fact that rate of depression has been long known to be predominantly female. For example, lifetime prevalence of major depression is 21 percent in women versus 12 percent in men. Similarly, lifetime prevalence of dysthymia* is 8 percent in women versus 5 percent in men. Furthermore, there are specific risk periods for women: the premenstrual phase of the ovarian cycle, the immediate postpartum period, and perimenopause.

*Definition: a chronic disturbance of mood involving a depressed mood for most of the day, for more days than not, for at least two years. Sometimes called depressive neurosis. It has been described by individuals as "sad or down in the dumps." Symptoms are: poor appetite or overeating, insomnia, low energy or fatigue, low self-esteem, poor concentration, and feelings of hopelessness.

In this text, Dr. Arlene Huysman places an important spotlight on one of these areas: mood swings after childbirth. She follows through in this text an area of currently limited understanding that despite its mysterious nature, receives much media attention due to the extreme, violent results of the mood changes in some cases. A mother who kills her children—and then lies about it—goes beyond the comprehension of most people. For the lay reader, Dr. Huysman carefully outlines the diagnostic background and significance of chemistry and hormones, and then proceeds to lay a groundwork for clearly understanding the often bizarre events that can occur during the postpartum period. In following her carefully laid foundation, she leads the reader to logically trace the development of depression, the onset of mania, and the role played by significant others.

As a practicing psychologist with extensive background in the treatment of mood disorders, Dr. Huysman is in a unique position to assess this aspect of these conditions, which all fall into the mood disorder category. Her background includes participation in the earliest lithium administration at University of Miami soon after its introduction—a breakthrough in management and prophylaxis. This was followed by years of collaboration with distinguished local psychiatrists in the pursuit of knowledge of the etiology and treatment of bipolar disorder. We have collaborated in many difficult cases in which her understanding of the personal and family dynamics have been a key factor in patient recovery.

A Mother's Tears is written by an individual who both has the background and experience to put its subject into perspective for all readers, no matter what that person's source of interest may be. The reader is not left hanging either; Dr. Huysman provides direction for the reader who may need help for herself or someone she knows.

This book is eminently readable—it holds the viewer's attention. One might think that such a text would be dry and boring, with lots of statistics. Although the requisite scientific basis is present, the text, quite the contrary, keeps the reader alert and focused by using many examples from national media and local cases. Thus, Dr. Huysman proceeds from the theory to data to application. The language is clear, precise, and stimulating. In fact, *A Mother's Tears* is difficult to put down. For this reason, *A Mother's Tears: Understanding the Mood Swings that Follow Childbirth* is an important and unique contribution to the literature on postpartum depression and mood disorders.

Paul J. Goodnick, M.D.
Director, Mood Disorders Program
Professor of Psychiatry and Behavioral Sciences
University of Miami School of Medicine
Miami, Florida
February 12, 1998

AUTHOR'S NOTE

THE OBSERVATIONS and characteristics I describe in
A Mother's Tears, in an effort to illuminate what is and is not known
about postpartum depression and progressive postpartum depression, are based on my experiences.

However, the details of people and places have been changed or
combined to create a composite of many patients, not only of mine,
but those of my colleagues as well.

Except for the headline cases—those having appeared in the
national and local newspapers, television shows, and magazines—
the names I have used in *A Mother's Tears* are fictitious to protect the
privacy of the patients and their families. Similarly, quotations have
been changed somewhat to disguise the many women who have
shared their experiences with me.

Many of the same characteristics appear in women with postpartum depression; therefore they may sound familiar in the descriptions and interviews throughout the book.

Arlene M. Huysman, Ph.D.
May 1998

Forget that you once loved them, that of your body
they were born. For one short day, forget your
children: afterwards, weep. Though you kill them,
they were your beloved....

—Euripides, *Medea*

PREFACE

Which of us doesn't know and marvel at that incredible Super Mom who rarely sleeps, has tremendous energy, works for hours taking care of the children while holding a part-time job, contributing time to charities, getting to bed at 1:00 AM and up again six, cleaning the house by seven, before taking the kids to school? But what about her sudden disappearance or unexplained illness, while the rest of the family has to take over the household and she withdraws, seems to be sick physically and depressed for months on end? What about the mental problems in her family that were always hidden? The uncle who spent his entire life in the hospital; the cousin who died mysteriously in her early twenties—it was rumored by some that she had hanged herself?—Ronald R. Fieve, M.D., *Moodswing*[1]

AS I EMBARKED on the writing of this book, I recalled the time of my own daughter's birth. My pregnancy had proceeded well and my baby, Pam, was healthy and certainly the most beautiful child ever born. The house was ready for us to return from the hospital. My husband was overjoyed with the baby. Everything was perfect.

Yet, if everything was so perfect, why was I crying uncontrollably? Why did the hospital room seem colorless and flat? Why wasn't I happy on what should have been the proudest day of my life? Why was I, in fact, miserable? I did not want to go home, or anywhere else. Suicide hovered in my mind as I wondered what I had gotten into.

When my doctor came by my hospital room for a routine check, he found me shedding tears of anguish.

"The nurse I hired cannot come to help me now," I choked, turning to him for comfort and help. His stinging response still wounds.

"Do you know what you remind me of, my dear? You make me think of a Toulouse-Lautrec painting."

I continued to cry. Toulouse-Lautrec meant nothing to me.

"You remind me of the painting of two well-dressed dowagers agonizing over what to order from the menu of a chic Parisian café. On the other side of the window, on the street, is a hungry tramp looking into his hand which holds only two coins. Not enough even for a cup of coffee," the doctor continued.

"You are like those women," he said.

The doctor left. "Of course he's right," I thought to myself. "I deserve to be humiliated. I am no better than those silly French women." I cried harder. I was so confused and distraught that I mistook my doctor's self-assurance for God's truth. And when my husband came to pick me up, I knew better than to share my feelings again.

The following day we took Pam home. I continued to hide my feelings of despair, even though they continued to reoccur in times of stress. But I did not have a genetic predisposition to depression, so the condition abated on its own. I know now that I was one of the lucky ones.

For numerous others, however, the condition not only continues, it worsens. And as the first-hand accounts below by mothers who suffered from postpartum depression (PPD) indicate, in some of the untreated cases, dire, sometimes even fatal, consequences are the end result.

One mother, a twenty-four-year-old waitress and student, confessed, "Ever since I brought the baby home I was living in a fog. I was so confused I did not know if it was day or night. When my husband ran the shower I thought it was raining inside the house. When a voice told me that my baby was a demon, I knew God had spoken to me. When God said, 'Smother the demon,' I did."

A twenty-two-year-old aspiring actress and new mother mumbled, "I did not hate the baby, I hated myself and nobody listened to me."

A twenty-seven year-old law school graduate and new mother of twins stated, "I was in a fog. Everything was flat and colorless. I knew my husband did not love me, my babies did not love me. How could they love me? I was worthless. Changing a diaper was beyond me. My husband reassured me and went on expecting me to snap out of it."

A thirty-two-year-old mail order executive cried, "Everyone said I was the perfect mother. I tended the house, my business, and my husband twenty-four hours a day. I did not sleep or eat anything besides Rice Krispies. The baby thrived without me. Luckily my mother and sister loved to watch little Tommy. They changed and bathed him until my husband got home. No one noticed that I kept as far away as possible from Tommy. Every time he cried I felt like lightening was striking me and tearing me apart. I was an unnatural mother."

A twenty-five-year-old travel agent explained: "My husband and I brought our baby home from the hospital. I was relieved when the nurse insisted we strap Tonia into a car seat. I was not comfortable holding her. All I wanted to do was sleep. When I did, I dreamed I was being pursued by a monster with my father's smile. In the dreams I stumbled and fell into the bassinet that held my screaming baby. When I awoke and looked at Tonia, I felt she was purposely in my way. She knew I was a loser and hated me for it. That is why she cried all the time."

THIS BOOK IS WRITTEN to educate and comfort women concerning the normal hormonal changes which take place after the birth of a baby. It attempts to help women understand the origins of behaviors and feelings previously thought to be psychologically based.

The book is also designed as a primer on the subject of postpartum depression and elucidates the treatments which are available for most victims of this condition. As the numerous comments above by mothers who experienced postpartum depression reveal, the feelings of the women who have suffered the effects of this mysterious disease—postpartum depression—are as dramatic as their unfathomable actions. This book explores the causes and effects of postpartum depression, as well as measures of prevention. It will serve as a valuable educational tool for women—both before and during pregnancy, and after the birth—and for their families.

Many myths have been perpetuated about postpartum depression, just as similar misconceptions have passed for truth about menopause.

If women know the truth and where to find help, they can benefit from early detection of the disorder. Many women suffer in silence, condemning themselves over their own bizarre thoughts or behavior. They have felt alone, frightened, misunderstood, and reviled for their feelings. They are ashamed.

These women need to know about the miraculous and often confusing developments in their hormonal systems where chemicals are perpetuating a tidal wave of physical and emotional changes.

A woman typically first becomes aware of mood changes before and/or during her menstrual cycle with reactions such as anger, irritability, or an increase in energy. If she had a predisposition to moodiness, it might become worse during the premenstrual cycle. Pregnancy also produces dramatic changes in a woman's hormonal balance.

Many of the chemical changes which are natural in the life cycle and monthly cycle of women have been ignored and have deterred women, the medical profession, and society in general from gaining the insight that would preempt catastrophe. Though millions of women suffer debilitating symptoms during these cycles, recognition and help has been a long time coming. The treatment available for these women corrects chemical and hormonal imbalance and alleviates pain and suffering, leaving them with the ability to feel "normal."

For example, premenstrual syndrome (PMS) can be treated with a number of new medications and approaches; symptoms from menopause can also be treated with a variety of approaches, including the addition of estrogen, as a replacement for the loss of naturally occurring hormones. Women do not have to suffer the same distressing symptoms that they did years ago.

Of course, not all women need or want to be treated for what they consider to be normal functions of the body. But the truth is that a percentage of women do need and want treatment and alleviation of symptoms.

Eighty percent of women who give birth experience some form of a postpartum upset. Of these women, between 20 and 40 percent report emotional disturbance or cognitive dysfunction or both. A smaller percentage suffer severe and even debilitating symptoms. Among this group there appears to be a persistent increase in the incidence of psychiatric illness, especially affective (mood) disorders in the two years following childbirth. Still another group develops a lifelong progressive condition, which I call *progressive postpartum depression* (PPPD). It is my belief that it is this long-term, progressive, and most importantly, treatable, condition that is the source of many of the filicide cases appearing in news headlines nationwide.

It was one of these headline cases, in fact, that served as the initial catalyst for my professional focus on postpartum depression: the now well-known case of Susan Smith, the South Carolina woman who killed her two sons. When I first read the story in *The New York Times*, I was stunned, and could not get the case out of my mind for days. As a woman and mother, I cringed. As a professional, the case appalled me. I felt so deeply about the problem that I decided I would talk to as many of today's 'Susan Smiths' as I could find in the hopes of gaining first hand-knowledge into the source of these violent outcomes. Those interviews, combined with information from current medical literature and from my own practice, form the basis of this book.

A Mother's Tears has absolutely nothing to do with innocence, guilt, or the judicial system. It has everything to do with an illness that in some cases, precipitates a bizarre set of behaviors, resulting in actions which then involve the judicial system. Once postpartum depression and progressive postpartum depression have been recognized sufficiently to insure that all mothers' suffering will be identified and treated, then a determination can be made as to how the judicial system might handle the unusual crimes that sometimes result when these conditions go undetected.

SOME OF THE FRIGHTENING statistics on child abuse only confirm my hypothesis and underscore the urgency of the situation nationwide. A recent Department of Justice study of 8,063 homicides in urban areas found that parents were charged in 57 percent of the murders of children under the age of 12. The U.S. Department of Health and Human Services calculates that in 1992 about 1,100 children died from abuse or neglect. Charles Ewing, a law and psychology professor at the State University of New York at Buffalo, estimates that only half the country's abuse deaths are uncovered.

Ninety percent of these deaths involve children under one year of age. It is my opinion that in a great percentage of these incidents, the mother of the abused or murdered child was clinically depressed and was suffering from postpartum or progressive postpartum depression.

No individual practitioner knows everything on the subject of mood disorders, and I am no exception. But I do know one thing for certain: No illness can be properly treated if it has not been correctly diagnosed. I also know that a mother's natural instinct is to nurture and protect her children.

I am a practicing clinical psychologist. My specialty is mood disorders, which can take the form of manic-depression. My years of experience and training as a clinical psychologist have given me the foundation I need to interpret the data and the literature on mothers who kill their children. My experience as a woman and a mother up against an unresponsive medical profession has given me the drive to study this disturbing question of human behavior.

During the writing of this book, I came to realize that previously, in my practice, I had adopted a "don't ask, don't tell" attitude about postpartum depression, just as many of my colleagues have. I had neglected to probe my female patients about the onset of their symptoms and when the first sign of depression occurred. Certainly I had always asked the question of when the depression began, but their answers did not connect my thinking to postpartum depression.

The cases of postpartum depressions that many of my colleagues and I treat have a common set of symptoms. They are always accompanied by shame and denial—by the mothers as well as by their partners and other significant family members. And yet there is no protocol among practitioners for addressing these symptoms. I believe that many of my colleagues need to have a clearer understanding of the mother who kills in order to save children, mothers, and society from similar tragedies.

IN THE COURSE OF researching this book, I found shelves and shelves of popular books on conception, pregnancy, birth, and everything concerned with what the expectant mother should know. There were books on nursing, on naming, on toddlers, on toilet training, on parenting, and on every aspect of early childhood development. Nowhere in all these volumes did I find literature specifically on the new mother. The only references were to regaining her pre-pregnancy figure with diet and exercise.

Where was the comprehensive literature on a possible serious depression after the birth of a child? There were only some vague statements like "you may feel angry or depressed. If you do, just speak to your doctor about it," or "these feelings will probably last the first few weeks." But where was the advice to mothers whose depressions continued? How was an "at risk" woman to know that she might be in for a very long and possibly tragic experience?

A prominent gynecologist I know shrugged it off as "something women learn about in prenatal classes." Most pediatricians usually only deal with problems of the baby, and most other health care clinicians tend to overlook postpartum symptoms. Even my colleagues—psychologists, psychiatrists, social workers, and mental health counselors—address the problem only when the family becomes affected in some way. To make matters worse, most of the existing literature is written for the doctor and not for the expectant mother.

One solution to this problem, of course, lies in the training of these clinicians. In all the cases which I have treated, those mothers who have been admitted to a hospital or been treated on an outpatient basis, have averted tragedy. The cases of filicide and/or extreme abuse we read about in the headlines, for the most part, probably have not been referred to or noticed by a professional who might have averted the outcome.

This book is based on theoretical thinking, careful study of headline cases, descriptions of cases that some of my colleagues and I have treated, and interviews with women who have already suffered the consequences of insufficient knowledge regarding their condition. I hope *A Mother's Tears* will serve as an educational tool for the general public, much as books on pregnancy, child rearing, and other family issues do.

There will be those who will disagree with my concept of progressive postpartum depression as a cause of many of the child murders by mothers. At the very least, I hope the disagreement and controversy it causes will provoke more curiosity about the subject and that the statistics, the histories, and the outcomes, will speak for themselves.

I would welcome further research, study, and interest in this area by other clinicians in order to validate my findings.

The information provided by my patients has convinced me that until the medical/psychological establishment gains a fuller understanding of postpartum depression, the tragedy will not end. Prevention through early detection is the answer.

1 | WHAT IS POSTPARTUM DEPRESSION?

> We know little about PMS [premenstrual syndrome]; we know less about postpartum depression, which in its mildest form affects an estimated 70 to 80 percent of all women following the birth of a child. From 10 to 20 percent of new mothers experience a full blown clinical depression. A far smaller number, approximately one in one thousand, develop a postpartum depressive psychosis.—Mark S. Gold, M.D., with Lois B. Morris, *The Good News About Depression: Cures and Treatments in the New Age of Psychiatry* [2]

WHAT IS TERMED "new baby blues" typically occurs within two weeks of delivery. In a mother without risk factors, it dissipates within weeks. But if this episode lasts two to three months, it can be considered postpartum depression. In order to gain a deeper insight into postpartum depression and the potential problems that may result from it, it is essential to have an understanding of the numerous changes a woman goes through during the pregnancy itself. For the nine months after conception the mother's body is transformed physiologically, biochemically, and psychologically to accommodate the development of the growing child within her.

Even prior to the awareness of the pregnancy, the mother has experienced pronounced changes in her body: she has missed several months of menstrual periods, has had morning nausea, and her breasts have swollen and become tender. During the early months of pregnancy, she has to urinate frequently because of pressure from the enlarging uterus on the bladder. She feels tired and drowsy. Her appetite changes and often she begins to dislike foods that she had previously enjoyed. She feels heaviness in the pelvic area. She may be subject to vomiting (sometimes severe) and to pulling pains in the sides of the abdomen as the growing uterus stretches the round muscles and ligaments that help support it.

As the pregnancy progresses, most of these symptoms may subside at the same time that dozens of other anatomic and physiologic changes occur. The uterus continues to enlarge, pushing the diaphragm upward, resulting in labored breathing. Even the external genital structures, breasts, and other organs and tissues undergo change.

Changes in the body continue after delivery of the baby, due largely to the greatly increased levels of the hormones estrogen and progesterone in the woman's blood. I'm sure most women are aware of the many outward manifestations of pregnancy, but are not really cognizant of the internal changes. The endocrine system, which is involved in every one of a woman's transitions—including menstruation, pregnancy, parturition (childbirth), postpartum, and menopause—controls various biochemical secretions. These may profoundly affect a woman's physiologic and psychological condition.

The endocrine system is comprised of three parts known as the hypothalamic-pituitary-adrenal axis. The two most prevalent endocrine secretions, measurable by blood levels, are estrogen and progesterone. Estrogens are a group of hormones that primarily influence the female reproductive tract. The major sources of estrogen are the ovaries and the placenta. These secretions also affect the vagina, fallopian tubes, uterus, and mammary glands. Progesterone is a hormone secreted by the female reproductive system that functions mainly to regulate the condition of the inner lining of the uterus. Usually the action of progesterone is accompanied by the activity of estrogen. During pregnancy it also stimulates development of the glands in the breasts that are responsible for milk production.

Other changes in the woman's body involve the cardiovascular and lymphatic systems which address the increasing needs of the growing baby and of the mother's own tissues. These throw an added burden onto the mother's heart. Since the heart actually undergoes a change in position during pregnancy, blood pressure and pulse rate are also affected.

The changes in the lymphatic vessels may cause swelling in the woman's legs. Her senses of taste and smell alter because of changes in the gastrointestinal tract. The intestines, liver, bladder, urinary tract, and kidneys also are involved in the new mother's biological metamorphosis.

As the entire metabolic system changes, weight becomes an issue. The woman may gain anywhere from ten to fifty pounds, which adds stress to her skeletal system.

Given that all these chemical, hormonal, and body changes take nine months to occur, the body has time to adjust to this gradual metamorphosis. However, the whole process culminates in the extreme physical exertion of the actual birth, aptly termed 'labor.' Even with a Caesarean section, the mother must heal from the trauma of surgery.

However, after the birth, every one of these systems that has undergone nine months of continual change now rapidly and dramatically transforms again. In addition to the physical changes, the new mother must simultaneously heal from the birth process, and deal with sleep deprivation, the engorgement of her breasts, lactation and nursing, the continuing physical and emotional needs of her other children, and the physical, emotional, and sexual needs of her husband or partner.

For women with any degree of genetic susceptibility to mood instability, the rapid hormonal adjustment, in addition to all the other factors, broadens her vulnerability to a bipolar illness, also known as manic-depressive illness.

There are also numerous environmental changes taking place in the new mother's life. A new baby, certainly a stranger in the home, brings with it a new schedule, a new element in the relationship between mother and partner and between mother and the home. The new stranger demands attention day and night, causing sleeplessness, as well as anxiety over all the new things any mother must learn quickly and adapt to immediately. Unless there is a very strong support system in place—mate, family, friends, paid helpers, or the like—the woman can lapse into a state of chaos and shock. Coupled with all the biochemical and hormonal changes, her task becomes Herculean. Imagine then having a predisposition to depression, anxiety, or suicide by virtue of genetics.

Many of the physiological and biochemical events that take place after the birth can explain a mother's dramatic changes of mood. But without a rare understanding of the inner workings of her own state of body and mind, during the time of pregnancy and after, a woman is not likely to know that there is, in fact, scientific and medical evidence of the changes with which a new mother must cope.

In one study, doctors measured estrogen and progesterone in women who had psychiatric symptoms, obstetric or medical complications, marital, or socioeconomic problems. They monitored blood samples at two- or three-day intervals for up to ten weeks postpartum. They found a correlation between irritability and higher pre-delivery estrogen levels. The greater the progesterone drop the more likely subjects were to rate themselves as depressed; they were also less likely to report sleep disturbances. In contrast, the lower the estrogen level, the more likely subjects were to report sleep disturbances.[3]

Though many of the studies have insufficient data to establish a diagnosis of depression, most clinicians agree that there is sufficient implication regarding physiological and biochemical events in postpartum psychiatric disorders, primarily involving the endocrine system. One of the best-known chemicals associated with mood disorders is called cortisol. This secretion has been and can be tested to determine depressive disorders.

The variety of biochemical changes taking place in a woman's system during her menses, pregnancy, post-pregnancy, and menopause involve, in addition to estrogen and progesterone, cortisol, prolactin,* and tryptophan.** These chemicals rise and fall throughout the cycles we describe. How, therefore, could changing levels not effect a woman's mood, as evidenced by such signs as tearfulness, depression, irritability, and anxiety?

Until now, postpartum depression has been associated only with the first six weeks after birth. And it is true that this early appearance of the illness occurs most frequently and is the easiest to diagnose and treat. But in other cases in which symptoms remain serious after the first six weeks, it could be said that a woman has been suffering from a serious postpartum depression since the time of the birth.

Consider the following case of one new mother whose name I've changed to protect her privacy:

Ariel and her husband were delighted when Ariel discovered she was pregnant. Her pregnancy and the birth proceeded normally.

---

*Definition: a pituitary hormone required for lactation.
**Definition: a dietary amino acid which is a precursor for brain serotonin, a neurotransmitter in the modulation by estrogen and progesterone.

When their new daughter, Lydia, was born, Ariel described herself as "the happiest woman on the planet." However, her happiness did not last long.

Within one week of her daughter's birth, Ariel began to feel depressed. Nothing she did either for herself, her husband, or the baby seemed to go right, and nothing her husband or her own mother said or did for her helped her feel any better about being a mother. Ariel's obstetrician advised the family not to worry. He told them that she had nothing wrong with her except for a commonplace case of "the OB Blues." At first, they all thought the doctor was right. Ariel began to feel better. Her mother, who had been staying with them, returned home, and her husband stopped feeling that he had to call every hour to check on Ariel and the baby.

But within a month, Ariel's depression returned—and this time it was worse. Her husband came home at the end of the work day to find the house dark, Ariel in bed, and the baby crying in the crib, unattended. He immediately called his mother-in-law for help.

Even with her mother's return and the extra attention now being given again to the baby, Ariel kept slipping into what her husband called her "trance." Eventually, even though she would improve for periods, the depressions continued.

Nine months after Lydia was born, Ariel called her husband at work, her voice barely a whisper. She told him he had to come home and watch Lydia. When he arrived, Ariel was emotionally and physically undone. Her husband was witnessing his wife turn from the loving and sweet woman he had known into a shadow of herself. He began to admit that he felt she no longer loved him or the baby.

Ariel whispered that she had to go to the hospital. Although her husband recognized the seriousness of her condition, he felt restrained by the stigma of a possible mental condition—what would his family and co-workers say? It was the next thing Ariel said that moved him to action. "Please, please, don't let me hurt our baby," she implored her husband.

Ariel may have saved her child's life. She certainly saved her marriage. She was diagnosed with a mood disorder and immediately put on an aggressive course of anti-depressant medication. Within weeks she was back home.

Ariel's recovery was not instantaneous, but it was continual. She needed and got counseling to help her shed the guilt for the thoughts and feelings she felt toward her baby daughter and her husband.

On Lydia's fourth birthday, Ariel learned that she was pregnant again. She, her husband, and her doctor approached this pregnancy carefully, but without fear.

Ariel's unusual insight into her own dangerous state of mind is exceptional. Not everyone can recognize this illness or its dangerous possibilities. It most often falls to others to identify the symptoms.

SIGNS OF POSTPARTUM DEPRESSION

Among the most recognizable signs of this illness are severe anxiety, panic attacks, spontaneous crying long after the usual duration of "baby blues" (i.e., three-seven days postpartum), lack of interest in her new infant, and insomnia (more likely to manifest as difficulty falling asleep than as early morning awakening, a common symptom of depression).

Other signs and symptoms of postpartum depression (also called PPD) which are sometimes only observable by family, friends, or clinicians, include:

- Complaints by the mother to someone—her husband, mother, or perhaps even her obstetrician—of such unremarkable and vague symptoms as "not being well."

❥ Continual complaints by the mother to other doctors of not sleeping or of having nightmares.

❥ Complaints by the mother of feeling irritable.

❥ Chronic irritability by the mother which provokes marital problems and family conflict.

❥ Thoughts of suicide that begin to pervade the mother's mind.

❥ Episodes of hyperactivity that begin with insomnia and increased energy.

❥ Episodes in which the new baby or a sibling may come to the attention of a pediatrician because of neglect or abuse.

SOME PROFESSIONALS MIGHT treat these complaints and symptoms strictly as psychological problems. No one may be aware that these inappropriate thoughts, feelings, and behaviors are symptoms of a medical problem.

No two people experience mood disorders in the same way or to the same degree. To extend the analogy of a common cold, one person may have sniffles and a light cough, while another may develop pneumonia and be hospitalized. Symptoms that lead to pneumonia start with the sniffles and a light cough. Not all sniffles and coughs lead to pneumonia.

Dr. Barbara Parry of the University of California School of Medicine, San Diego, characterizes postpartum depression as melancholia,* neurasthenia,** and severe insomnia*** appearing within six

---

*Definition: marked by suicidal thinking and behavior, mental and physical slowing, physical complaints, self-denigration, guilt, confusion, indecision, marked fatigue, ruminative thinking, morbid obsessions and irrational fears.
**Definition: a heaviness of arms and legs.
***Definition: an inability to sleep.

months of childbirth and lasting from six to nine months. She states its incidence is ten to fifteen percent. She reports that while postpartum psychosis* is far less common, with an incidence of 0.1 percent, it is far more dangerous. Four percent of women who develop this disorder kill their children.

One reason many deaths (infanticides) have not been associated with postpartum depression is that the cases involved not only babies, but also older children. Such cases involving older children have forced some of us to consider that postpartum depression, untreated, may continue for years after birth. If so, the only logical conclusion is that the depression is progressive and was the result of a biochemical imbalance triggered originally by the birth and exacerbated by an event such as a severe loss, a rejection, a divorce, poverty, or the loss of a job or a parent.

The concern for women in conjunction with having children, therefore, is not simply postpartum depression, but the long-term and potentially destructive effects of progressive postpartum depression (PPPD).

The addition of the word *progressive* brings the entire syndrome into a framework wherein the birth event triggers a long-term and serious illness, a psychopathology, which is definable, treatable, and controllable—but only once it is recognized as such. This means that the medical profession should be capable of dealing with the disorder once it has been acknowledged as an illness.

Suicidal thoughts very often accompany postpartum depressions, possibly as a defense mechanism against harming the child. Most clinicians will agree that people who commit suicide are not in their "right" minds. Similarly, mothers who kill their own children can be considered to be mentally unbalanced. The depression has affected

---

*Definition: clouding of consciousness, disorientation, perplexity, and visual hallucinations.

their cognition (defined as what you have learned and what you know intellectually), and may cause them to 'unlearn' or temporarily forget those moral statutes that they have learned and that we all take as a given in society—that murdering one's own child is an unnatural act and out of the realm of anything we have learned in our development.

One of the theories on suicide gives us a great deal of insight into the occurrence of the postpartum phenomenon. Sigmund Freud asserted that suicide is an aggressive act. I believe this is true in more than one sense: it is self-assault aiming at self-punishment, self-destruction, or the destruction of something that is, or ought to be, of value to others.

Freud also believed that suicide should not be explained as an act of aggression against the self, but rather as an act of hostility directed against others. These same concepts of aggression and of destroying something of value that Freud used to try to understand and explain suicide relate similarly to the harming of a child—the most precious of all possessions. Though it is the child who is killed, infanticide can still be regarded as an aggressive attempt by the mother at self-assault and self-punishment. In other words, since most mothers view their children as extensions of themselves, killing the baby is a way of killing part of themselves. Simultaneously, such an act can also be regarded as a hostile message from the mother directed at others in the family who have not recognized the depression the mother is experiencing as a serious problem.

The following case about a patient who is a professional therapist aptly illustrates the strong connection between suicidal thoughts, behavior, and postpartum depression. She was initially reluctant to relate her story because of the stigma she feared would reflect on her professionally. She learned of the story from her grandmother who told it to her when she was a young adult. It had always been kept a secret in the family.

It seems that the woman's mother, who became pregnant on her honeymoon, gave birth to her when she was hardly an adult herself. Because the family did not approve of the marriage, she returned from the hospital stay to a small apartment in Philadelphia with no family support and a husband in economic crisis.

"My mother must have been extremely frightened as she tried to care for me. She must have been unaware of how depressed and hopeless she felt about our future," the woman explained. One morning her mother carefully placed towels around the openings of all the doors and windows and turned on the gas stove. The mother and infant were found semi-conscious, barely in time to save their lives.

Many of the women who have committed a crime against their children speak of hoping to "save" the child from a life of misery. The implication of this paradox is that despite their acts of violence, these women desire their babies just as much as the women who do not have a predisposition to the illness. They have the same capacity to love and nurture their babies as other women. Despite this fact, however, we can clearly surmise that one must be very ill to entertain and rationalize any thought process that justifies or precipitates violence directed at a child.

Dewey Cornell, a clinical psychologist at the University of Virginia, affirms the notion that suicide and postpartum depressions often go hand in hand, asserting, "Most typically [a female act of violence against her children occurs] ...in context of a woman who is severely depressed and may also be suicidal." Indeed, this seems to be the case often. It is not hard to link a mother's suicidal ideation with psychosis or postpartum depressions. Susan Smith, the South Carolina woman who made headlines when it was discovered that she killed her two sons, for example, had not only thought of suicide, she had attempted it several times.

Manic* symptoms, as opposed to depressive symptoms, are another postpartum manifestation and are predominant in 40 percent of cases. Some women may develop these symptoms, marked by extreme hyperactivity, elation, poor judgment, sleeplessness, and agitation. The mania may be a result of genetic predisposition and is usually followed by a depression.

A mother may experience an episode with symptoms of either mania or depression within days or weeks after giving birth. It is likely that this episode will be of limited duration. It can last hours, days, or weeks. The mother usually will "recover" or seem to and return to feeling normal, then may actually lapse into a depression.

Mania may be described in the case of 35-year-old Deborah Turner of Chicago who hurled her son, Tyler, to his death through a closed, eighth floor window when he wouldn't stop crying.[4] She had been distraught, and had not slept or eaten for three or four days. Her sister, Edwina Banks, said Deborah was under stress from rearing her children—ages 8, 12, and 13—alone. She was facing eviction. Now she also had to care for her 16-month-old son, Tyler.

Deborah was jailed without bail and Edwina bemoaned: "What she did was madness. She didn't have to toss her flesh and blood out the window. All he wanted her to do was hold him." Wearing only a diaper, Tyler landed on the muddy ground outside an urban housing project. Her sister said, "I don't know what made her snap."

Deborah had apparently raised her other children without having any previous contact with the State Department of Children and Family Services.

Deborah was visiting Edwina when she killed Tyler. "She was acting all distraught," said Edwina, "walking and saying things that didn't make sense."

---

*Definition: a form of mental disorder, marked by great excitement.

Edwina continued, "I said 'Deborah, try to eat something' ...She got up, and she carried the baby into the bedroom." Then, Edwina and others in the apartment heard glass breaking. She rushed into the room and saw the shattered window.

"She was standing there by the window," Edwina recalled. "I asked her 'Deborah, why did you do that?' ...She couldn't say anything. So I just slapped her as hard as I could, then ran downstairs to check on the boy."

Deborah's 13-year-old son, Demetri Turner, said his mother had never been abusive before. And Edwina Banks said her sister had always been a good mother. This, in my experience, is a clear cut case of postpartum psychosis, manifested as a mania.

WE EXPECT THAT a simple and time-limited postpartum depression will abate on its own or be treated in a timely fashion. The mother with *progressive* postpartum depression (PPPD), however, does NOT recover without treatment. She merely experiences a hiatus until her next episode. Subsequent episodes are very often triggered by rejections, separations, and losses, and recur throughout the woman's life. Usually the next episode is worse than the last. If this pattern goes unchecked, the mother will spiral into a cycle of illness that can destroy her life and her family.

When a mother is in the grip of this disease in its most serious form, she passes beyond reason. In place of the capable woman is one full of dread, rage, and confusion. She feels unloved and unlovable and loses her ability to distinguish right from wrong. She may hear voices in her head and be listening to them rather than the voices of her family. This is not a symptom of schizophrenia, but rather a reflection of her own obsessive thinking. Death may become a preoccupation. She is in the throes of what feels like an unending despair.

SOCIETY'S VIEW OF MOTHERHOOD

It is contrary to the very experience of motherhood to hurt—let alone kill—a child, which, after all, begins as an extension of a woman's body and soul, a being whom she has given the breath of life. Every culture has its own particular view of motherhood which derive from experience and from legends, history, and literature.

Universally, motherhood is both a symbol—of creativity, birth, fertility, nurturance, and growth—and an experience that women have. Mothers have been depicted as everything from goddesses of fertility to the Virgin Mary. In most societies, mothers have been given an honored place. The Earth Mother is the eternally fruitful source of nourishment. All things come from her, return to her, and are nurtured by her. She gives birth from her womb and she nourishes all from her breasts. The symbol of the mother goddess emphasizes her maturity. She is the protector and nourisher of the innocent child and in our mind's eye we see her as a figure holding the babe in her arms.

Of course, geographically and culturally we know this is not an accurate picture of all mothers everywhere and all the time. There are also the mothers in literature who have killed their children for politics, love, money, jealousy, and power. Depression or insanity, however, are not usually seen as explanations for their actions.

Clarissa Pinkola Estés writes of some of the different kinds of mothers in her book, *Women Who Run with the Wolves*. Her approach, one of Jungian psychoanalytic theory, describes an external and an internal mother. According to Estés, the internal mother is: "[an] aspect of the psyche that acts and responds in a manner identical to a woman's experience in childhood with her own mother. This internal mother is made from not only the experience of the personal [biological] mother, but also from other mothering figures in our lives, as well as the images held out as the good mother and the bad mother in the culture at the time of our childhoods. "For most adults, if there was trouble with the mother once but no more, there is still a duplicate mother in the psyche who sounds, acts, and responds the same as in early childhood... the internal mother will have the same values and ideas about what a mother should look and act like, as those in one's childhood."[5]

Estés goes on to define the various roles of motherhood: the ambivalent mother; the collapsed mother; the child mother or the unmothered mother; and the strong mother, the strong child.

I believe, as Estés suggests, that, coupled with the hormonal changes after the birth of her child, the new mother mentally replays the old tapes of what her mother was like to her. If she was abused, beaten, terrorized, or abandoned, all these dynamics would be exaggerated when mixed with the postpartum depression. If, in fact, there was a history in her family of any of the traits you will learn about in subsequent chapters, the mother will be helpless to amend any behavior learned in her past.

Estés's unmothered mother in particular offers a good example of this tendency. According to Estés's description, she is fragile, she wishes to have babies, even though she may be unable to care for them, and she may be very young and innocent. Additionally, "she may be so physically dislocated that she considers herself unlovable even by a baby. She may have been so tortured by her family [and their genetic traits] and her culture that she cannot imagine herself worthy of touching the hem of the 'radiant mother' archetype that accompanies new motherhood."[6]

Estés's theory clearly points out the need for support by family members, her immediate society, her significant other, her clinician(s), etc. She goes on to say that the mother "is likely to suffer from naive presentments, lack of seasoning, and in particular a weakened instinctual ability to imagine what will happen one hour, one week, one month, one year, five years, ten years from now."

As the information in subsequent chapters will bear out, this link between family history of depression and other at-risk traits and a predisposition to postpartum depression is not a new phenomenon. There is ample evidence that this condition has afflicted women throughout the ages. For example, the 19th-century description of PPD in Charlotte Perkins Gilman's Victorian novella, *The Yellow Wallpaper* offers one of the most dramatic examples in literature of a postpartum depression. A fictionalized account of Gilman's own experience with PPD, *The Yellow Wallpaper* tells the story of a woman taken to the country by her husband, a physician, to recover from an unidentified malaise, a nervous fatigue that has overtaken her after the birth of her baby. However, his treatment, a perfect example of 19th-century attitudes toward women, results in her slow, steady decline into psychosis. Treating her like a child, he isolates her, placates her, and ignores her descriptions of her state of mind: "He [her husband] says no one but myself can help me out of it, that I must use my will and self control and not let any silly fancies run away with me."[7] Slowly, madness becomes her only freedom.

This description of a 19th-century woman's downward spiral into psychosis becomes more sobering in light of the fact that *The Yellow Wallpaper* was based on the real-life experiences of its author, Charlotte Perkins Gilman, who continued for the rest of her life to suffer the effects of her untreated postpartum depression. Elaine R. Hedges, in the Afterword of Gilman's book, writes that Gilman became "a mental wreck" within a month of giving birth to her daughter. From the time of her marriage Gilman wrote of feeling that "...something was going wrong.... A sort of gray fog drifted across my mind, a cloud that grew and darkened." She increasingly felt weak, sleepless, and was unable to work. Certainly this fore-shadowed her feelings after the birth: "There was a constant dragging weariness...Absolute incapacity. Absolute misery."[8]

Although both Gilman's husband and brother were physicians, her journey to insanity was trivialized and treated as temporary. The two men presumed and fully expected that her condition would abate on its own. They were wrong.

More distressing, however, is the fact that even though this true story occurred at the turn of the last century, attitudes towards women's postpartum behavior have scarcely changed.

2 | WHO IS AT RISK?

I know now that my family background makes me a prime candidate. My father was an alcoholic, which is common in families with manic-depression. And in 1980 my mother was diagnosed as having unipolar depression, the lows without the highs. Because she had that illness, she made choices and decisions that affected the way I grew up. The results of those choices plus my genetics made me very vulnerable.— from Chapter Three of *A Brilliant Madness: Living with Manic-Depressive Illness* by Patty Duke and Gloria Hochman[9]

THE RISK OF POSTPARTUM depression is highest in women over twenty-five years of age who have a history of mood instability. It is estimated that of these, 30 to 40 percent will have a postpartum episode. Also among those prone to PPD are genetically predisposed women, those with a family history of mood instability.

To help define and predict which women are at risk, it is necessary to know the medical and psychological history of the biological family. So much of the mother's state of mind, before and after the birth, will depend on her predisposition to a mood disorder. Behavior traits in a family offer clues to a genetic predisposition in a candidate.

Traits are not symptoms, but rather characteristics that are prevalent in a family prone to mood disorders. Studies show that people with mood disorders come from families in which mood disorders are the norm rather than a rarity. Pathology begets pathology. A thorough study of family history is essential in making the diagnosis of a predisposition towards progressive postpartum depression (PPPD).

Most of these characteristics will also have biological implications. However for the sake of simplicity, I will name and describe these traits, as well as the behaviors associated with them.

Foremost is a family history of suicide or a preoccupation with suicidal thoughts. There is a direct correlation for severe depressions in families where suicide or suicidal thoughts are also present. *Psychiatric Dictionary* describes suicide, defined as "the act of killing oneself," in detail as follows: "While it is believed by some that all suicides are psychotic, the more widely accepted view is that suicide can occur in any psychiatric disorder although the psychoses (depressions, including involutional psychoses, and schizophrenia) account for the majority of cases. Alcoholics also contribute a disproportionately high number of suicides among the non-hospitalized population.... The larger the family, the smaller the risk of suicide; when classified by marital status and family constellation, suicides are seen to be most frequent among those who are divorced. While some series indicate that almost all suicides have had a relative who committed suicide or otherwise met a violent, tragic, or dramatic death, not all writers agree on the prognostic significance of the presence or absence of such loss of a loved one.... Among the clinical depressions, those with prominent anxiety features, a feeling of losing ground, and/or a marked hypochondriacal* trend are

---

*Definition: somatic overconcern; morbid attention to the details of body functioning and/or exaggeration of any symptom, no matter how insignificant, including easy fatigue, physical and mental weakness, aches, pains, insomnia, and inadequate functioning of any organ or organic system of the body.

the most likely to make a suicide attempt.... Suicide often occurs when the patient seems to be recovering from an emotional crisis; approximately half occur within 90 days of such crisis... the dynamic elements often clearly operative in the depressed patient when he/she loses the object which he/she depends upon for narcissistic supplies."[10]

Although suicidal tendencies are known to exist in a variety of illnesses, there is a direct link between a depressed mother having suicidal thoughts and the harm she may do to herself or her children. These thoughts and behaviors have also been correlated with chemical imbalances, which are apt to appear after the birth of the child.

Countless women suffering from the misery of a postpartum depression have expressed their anguish by considering suicide. For this reason, as described in Chapter One, I believe that the mother who feels compelled to harm or destroy her child is acting out her desire to harm or to "do away" with herself. A history of suicide or suicidal preoccupation is usually present in the family history. Conversely, a mother's suicide can also be an attempt to keep herself from harming her child.

One tragedy that did not appear in the newspapers is typical of those that are passed off simply as random suicides. "Mother was depressed," said family members afterward, without anyone seeing the connection to the birth.

The couple in this case had been married ten years before Betty became pregnant in her late thirties. When she became pregnant, she and her husband, Herb, were both ecstatic. Betty was a beautiful, professional woman with a career in public relations. Her husband, Herb, was handsome, well-known in the community, and was a successful businessman.

Despite this seemingly ideal scenario, as soon as their lovely daughter was born, the situation at home began to change. Betty

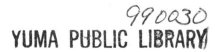

became nervous, suspicious that Herb "was seeing someone else." She complained that she didn't look as trim as before and that he had probably lost interest in her. Finally, overwrought and sleepless, she began to see a psychiatrist. He prescribed valium, a tranquilizer, to calm her down. It is important to recognize that many tranquilizers are depressants and addictive as well.

The more hysterical Betty became, the more mystified Herb grew and the more valiums Betty took. Luckily her mother was close by, so she took care of the baby.

Betty began to imagine that a woman was parked across the street from their house. And she was sure that this was the woman her husband was "seeing." She argued with Herb, argued with her mother, and felt her mother was not caring for her baby well. After a particularly terrible argument, she went upstairs, found a gun in the closet, and shot herself in the head. The baby was less than a year old.

SOME WOMEN AT RISK for progressive postpartum depression cannot be so recognized by others or by themselves by any outward sign. In these cases, knowing the family history, which may indicate a genetic predisposition to depression or to mood disorders, is vital.

Many times, women were adopted and are therefore unaware of their biological family history. Even in families with a complete family tree, depression and suicide have long carried a stigma. Many women have never been told about incidents in their own families. Even in close knit families, depression, alcoholism, or suicide may be "the elephant in the living room." The family members skirt around it and do not wish to acknowledge it. When family histories are not available, however, it is symptoms and signs that play an even more important role in diagnosing PPPD early on. Dr. Lynn Grush, associate director of the perinatal psychiatric clinical research program at

Massachusetts General Hospital, addresses the issue of an early diagnosis by saying that a potential postpartum depression would be easy to predict if the mother has had a history of depression or has had a diagnosis of bipolar disorder.

There is a great deal of similarity in the symptoms of these three conditions: 1) manic-depression (also called bipolar disorder), 2) postpartum depression (PPD), and 3) progressive postpartum depression (PPPD).

➤ Manic-depression is a genetic illness which manifests itself in its mildest form as mood instability and in its most extreme form as unpredictable mood swings ranging from mania to depression. This is a treatable biochemical imbalance.

➤ Postpartum depression, commonly called "maternity blues," is expected to ensue on the third day following delivery. Episodes of crying, sleeplessness, and anger come and go from 24 hours to a week and then lift.

➤ Progressive postpartum depression is a chronic series of symptoms that do not abate or seem to disappear but recur over the course of many weeks and even months, in some instances. These symptoms begin to increase in intensity and duration and will continue to reappear throughout the life of the mother. This is the condition that can evolve until it manifests itself in episodes so relentless and debilitating that they may result in tragedy.

THE GENERAL PUBLIC is usually unaware that those symptoms and/or a history of postpartum depressions, or depression of any kind in the family, are telling clues and should alert both the mother and family members to the potential danger.

Drs. Frederick K. Goodwin and Kay Redfield Jamison, in their comprehensive book *Manic-Depressive Illness,* point out the difficulty in differentiating genetic factors from true effects of the psychological and social impact of mothers with depressive disorders. While genetic factors when present certainly have an impact, Goodwin and Jamison feel that the behaviors of the mother may reflect her own learning from a similarly affected mother: "Clearly, it is not always easy to separate genetic factors, manifested in childhood or adolescent expressions of affective illness, from true effects of the psychological and social impact of bipolar parenting. Given the lack of complete penetrance, the combination of both environmental and genetic influences is not only the most probable but also the most conceptually interesting likelihood."[11]

Citing the work of Fabian and Donohue (1956), Rutter (1966), and Weissman and Paykel (1974), Goodwin and Jamison go on to emphasize that "many areas of childbearing are affected by maternal depression.... The difficulties experienced by depressed women in fulfilling their maternal roles has been researched extensively by Weissman and colleagues.... Weissman found that mothers, during an acute depressive episode, were less involved with their children, had impaired communication and increased friction, guilt, and resentment, [and] were overprotective, rejecting, irritable, and distant. The depressed women also reported greater degrees of discord with their children than with their friends, colleagues, or other members of their family. Increased hostility by depressed mothers toward their children has been observed by several investigators."

In small families, or families which may be scattered and/or estranged, as well as in cases of adoption, there may be difficulty in obtaining knowledge of the family history and recognizing the traits which may affect the family. This pertains to adopted adult children as well. In those cases clinicians must rely on clinical judgment and a keen eye and ear for events occurring during the postpartum period.

Other family traits* that spell out indications of a predisposition to psychotic or affective episodes and contribute to possible post-partum depression are: addiction to alcohol and/or drugs, family history of multiple marriages, compulsive gambling, poor judgment, indiscreet financial and sexual behaviors, impulsive or violent behavior, aggression, and inflated self-esteem or grandiosity. At risk are mothers from families that displayed one or more of the following traits: unstable and chaotic lifestyles, lack of empathetic regard for the rights of others, too much dependence on one another or too much independence from one another, extreme rigidity, compulsive behavior, and frequent bouts of rage.

Clinicians have known for a long time that most alcohol and drug abusers are attempting to self-medicate for other pre-existing conditions. In other words they drink or do drugs to either "pick themselves up" or "calm themselves down." Correspondingly, most of the recent literature accepts that people can have what is known as a "dual diagnosis"—two disorders at the same time—a mood disorder and an addiction problem.

Unfortunately, people who drink or abuse substances display behavior that makes it very difficult to pinpoint the underlying depression or mood disorder. Nevertheless, since child abuse and fil-icide have tended to go hand in hand with a history of alcohol and drugs in the mother or in the mother's family, it is important to determine the basis for the addiction—genetically.

In the case of Deborah Turner, described in Chapter One, police were investigating reports from neighbors and others that Turner had been smoking crack cocaine and drinking, even though her sister, Edwina, denied it. If the allegations about substance abuse were

---

*Definition: characteristic symptoms of a hereditary factor of those who have inherited the predisposition to any given illness.

true, Deborah's manic behavior was probably a combination of post-partum mania, alcohol, and drug use.

Other researchers and clinicians have made similar correlations. Steven J. Shea, Ph.D. and Geoffrey R. McKee, Ph.D, A.B.P.P., court appointed psychologists in *the State of South Carolina v. Susan Smith* case,[12] for example, find a host of common factors among the homicides of mothers who kill their children. During the writing of this book I had the opportunity to speak with one of these psychologists. Both are from the University of South Carolina School of Medicine. They have been involved not only in the Susan Smith case, but in those of other mothers who have killed their children and were being tried in South Carolina. They also presented their findings in August 1995 at the American Psychological Association's (APA) 103rd Annual Convention in New York City.

Shea and McKee's study describes 20 cases of mother-child fili-cide (including the Susan Smith case) comprising 26 deaths in which the women were ordered for pre-trial evaluations at the William S. Hall Psychiatric Institute for the State of South Carolina, a university-based forensic psychiatric hospital. Data collection began in 1986 and is ongoing, so that the number of cases is likely to increase.

In this study the women's ages ranged from 18 to 66 (adoptive mother) with an average age of 29.25 years. Forty-five percent of the women were white and 55 percent were African-American. The majority—65.0 percent—were legally married or in a common-law arrangement; of those, 42.9 percent described the relationship as abusive. The women reported 50 children in their care with 70 percent having two or more children. Of the fifty children, more that half—52.0 percent—became victims of maternal filicide.

The doctors conducting the study concluded that the majority of these women suffered from a diagnosable mental disorder. Most of the victims were less than 25 months old with 45 percent under one year, suggesting postpartum and/or adjustment issues. The data underscored the importance of early detection and treatment of mental illness in mothers. The risk to the child of abuse and death exists even though these mothers may have had no history of legal trouble.

Based on their findings in this study, Drs. Shea and McKee describe the typical characteristics of women who kill their children as:

> being the biological mother of the victim;
> being mentally ill at the time of the offense;
> killing a single child less than 25 months old;
> being legally married or in a common-law relationship;
> acting alone in their own home;
> having no history of prior arrest;
> being unemployed at the time of offense;
> being raised in a two-parent lower socioeconomic status background;
> having lower intelligence and educational level than average;
> having two or more children in their care.[13]

Their research and writing is very valuable in an arena where few researchers have correlated the common factors in these tragedies. However, while some of this data points to postpartum depression, my own practice has shown me that intelligence, educational, or socioeconomic status are not necessarily relevant. In my experience, not all women who kill their newborns are young, poor, uneducated, and socially isolated. On the contrary, they are from all walks of life, all cultures, economic classes, religions, and races. In fact, the recent rash of killing of newborns supports this premise. These women have come from middle-class and even affluent families. They have given birth at proms, at work, and at home, hiding their pregnancies while internally and psychologically suffering through nine months.

This is not to render the findings cited above useless. These factors, when present, may indeed serve as stressors that trigger episodes in women with a predisposition to mood disorders and we owe a great deal to clinicians like Shea and McKee who have added to the current body of literature on this subject and presented research that may help many more women get diagnosed. It is, however, important to note that these factors are not necessarily the *only* relevant characteristics. From the perspectives of both researchers and patients alike, it's exciting that there are more factors to uncover that may help with diagnosis and predictability. More research needs to be done and more clinicians should be sharing their findings and experience to add to the current pool of data.

THE PARENTS AS VICTIMS OF VIOLENCE
(Violence as a Predecessor)

❥ Eighty-five percent of childhood deaths from abuse and neglect are systematically misidentified. Over half the children who die are from families who have never been investigated by child protective service agencies.[14]

ACCORDING TO A NEWS ARTICLE in the April 26, 1995 *Los Angeles Times,* abuse and neglect in the home is the leading cause of death for young children in this country, exceeding deaths caused by urban gang wars, AIDS, polio, measles, accidental falls, choking on food, suffocation, drowning, or residential fires; yet public and professional attention is minimal in attempting to disseminate this information properly.

In my own experiences in treating families with cases of child abuse, negligence and even murder, I have found that there is almost always a history of acting out and violence in the mother's own family. In fact, violence in families with child abuse is much more the norm than the exception. The mother's own infancy and early childhood development play a major factor.

The incidence of family violence in Florida where I have my practice, for example, is disturbingly high. One person dies at the hands of a spouse, ex-spouse, or cohabitant approximately every three days. Further, a child who witnesses the perpetration of this violence becomes a victim, as she or he hears or sees it occurring, and is then traumatized by what he or she has seen—sometimes for life.

The same child is also at high risk of being the victim of physical abuse themselves—both by the parent who is perpetrating violence against their spouse, and, to a lesser extent, by the parent who is the victim. Fifty-seven percent of children under the age of twelve who are murdered, are murdered by a parent. Domestic abuse between adult partners is often accompanied by violence toward the children of the family. It is estimated that at least half of the men who abuse their female partners also abuse their children.[15]

In 1994 alone, 321 domestic homicides were reported in Florida; children accounted for one-quarter of the deaths. Most were under four years old and died from abuse or neglect. Attacks on them were often triggered by crying, problems with toilet training, and perceived disobedience. In an effort to deal with this pattern of domestic violence, the Florida Governor's Task Force on Domestic and Sexual Violence Against Women recommended a psycho-educational model similar to that used by the Domestic Abuse Program in Duluth, Minnesota. The philosophy underlying the recommendations were that "the primary focus of batterer's programs must be the safety of the battered women and her children." While this philosophy is a good start in addressing the problem of domestic violence, it completely overlooks the possibility that the mother may be a perpetrator of child abuse as well. Interestingly, the Task Force does not even mention postpartum depression as a possible factor or nor as a condition that can be either linked to, triggered by, or exacerbated by a pattern of domestic violence in a given family. Even as I was writing this book, I attended a workshop on domestic violence which totally omitted the topic of women's depression or postpartum depression as a contributing factor. This despite the fact that infants and small children were the victims in a large percentage of the domestic violence cases discussed.

Intervention programs that recognize postpartum depression as one of the possible sources of domestic violence would insure that women would come under the scrutiny of mental health professionals and get proper treatment. These programs would then provide the opportunity for caregivers to identify women who are depressed and unable to protect their children.

Some states are mandating that the primary purpose of their intervention programs shall be victim safety and the safety of the children, if present. I view this as a move in the right direction, since then those who work for victim safety programs would be able to insure some screening of women who are suffering from progressive postpartum depression.

It is accepted today that violence in families perpetuates itself in continued violence. Violent actions stem not only from a severely ill mental state, but also from a great deal of learned behavior. Most people raised in an environment of domestic violence (emotional or physical), tend to use the learning they received as a way to deal with life's stress. Domestic violence could not take place without affecting the entire family constellation. Obviously if violence is prevalent in the home, it will reach the children.

Experts also say a history of trauma—such as sexual victimization or physical abuse—can play into parents' impulses to kill their children, and to lie about it to themselves and others.

One case particularly bears this assertion out. Estella "Pixie" Good, 24, of Tampa, Florida, said that she was following her father's orders when she killed her 9-month-old son Skipper because he cried too much. Pixie also testified that her father, Eddie Lee Sexton, ordered Willie Sexton, her brother and Eddie Lee's son, to kill the baby's father, Joel Good, after he threatened to go to the police. Both bodies were found buried in Tampa-area state parks.

Pixie testified that her father had dominated her sexually and psychologically, and that he had been sexually abusing her since she was 17. He also fathered two of her children. Other family members stated that Sexton strapped Pixie's children to their beds in their own excrement, boiled a human fetus, and ordered a child to stand in a grave as part of a cult ceremony.

For her testimony, Pixie's sentence was reduced by half to six years for the strangulation of the child. Willie Sexton, Pixie's brother, was found incompetent to stand trial and is being treated at a state mental hospital. Eddie Lee Sexton, her father, was found guilty of first-degree murder and was sentenced to die in the electric chair. As horrific and unusual as this case is, it dramatically illustrates the perpetuation of abuse in the family system.

On a similar note, Susan Hiatt, the director of the Kempe National Center for the Prevention and Treatment of Child Abuse and Neglect in Denver, describes filicide as part of a larger web of neglect, stress, and abuse: "Generally, parents who kill their children tend to be under a lot of stress. The may be very young and may not be ready for the demands of parenthood. They are often socially isolated and do not have a large social network. They have also probably been victims of violence themselves."

A case in point is Amanda Wallace, age 31, who hanged her son, Joey, age 3, from a transom on April 19, 1993. Amanda had been abused at the hands of her own mother, and there were three boxes of Amanda's records from mental hospitals. She had been suicidal since age nine, had swallowed glass and nails, stabbed herself bloody with needles, and set fire to her bed. When she was not hurting herself, her mother was hurting her. This case and especially the death of little Joey could have been prevented had a history been taken by any health care professional in contact with Amanda Wallace.

It becomes more apparent that cases like Pixie's and Amanda's are not so unusual when we read that the level of violence in this country has reached public health crisis proportions, annually claiming the lives of at least 2,000 children and seriously injuring upward of 140,000 others. These statistics come from the U.S. Advisory Board on Child Abuse and Neglect.[16]

Following a 2 1/2-year nationwide study, the Board concluded that the level of fatal abuse and neglect is far greater than even experts in the field had previously realized. For example they found that the homicide rate among children under four years of age has hit a 40-year high.

The same report describes an alarming national environment of under-reported child abuse deaths. It also criticizes investigators, prosecutors, and medical professionals as being inadequately trained and conducting inconsistent autopsy practices: "Medical misdiagnosis is common, because in many states, determination of the causes of a child's death is made by a coroner with little or no medical training. Even highly trained medical examiners may not recognize the often subtle medical signs of child abuse and neglect. Moreover, there is still widespread reluctance among coroners and medical examiners to implicate a child's parents or involve themselves in criminal cases."[17] I add my voice to a statement in the report that the American public continues to regard child deaths as "rare curiosities."

My investigation has revealed that the same attitude exists in many other countries as well. Scientists in other countries, such as France, are also attempting to describe the condition in journals for professionals in an attempt to push their medical communities to recognize the frequency and severity of the disorder. A report from a French medical journal by F. Desseigne and J. Carrere reveals seven cases of mothers who killed their children. The report goes on to criticize the attitude of the medical establishment in France toward the problem:

"The depressive reactions should not be ignored [whether they occur before, during, or after a pregnancy] especially when Social Security [the health system in France] grants women with few allowances giving the patient the opportunity to be examined. It is a fact that those medical examinations are too quick and do not investigate the psychiatric past of the patient well enough in order to identify depressive antecedents.

"The obstetrician [in France] has [only] three visits. It would be helpful to allow mental health practitioners the same frequency of visits in order to prevent psychiatric troubles and eventually, to be able to prescribe contraceptive formulas if necessary."[18]

The authors of this report believe that throughout history, the view of this condition has not changed significantly; the behaviors are often perceived as evil rather than as manifestations of an illness. Given the natural tendency to view mothers as nurturers and caretakers, these acts are all the more difficult to understand.

The article points out how French psychiatrists are not even aware of many of these cases until they conduct special research. In France, when mother is successful at killing herself or her child, there is no investigation. Even though the French Department of Justice may have data on such cases, it is usually not examined. Unfortunately, reports like this one suggest the enormity of the problem and simultaneously indicate that the medical disregard for postpartum depression and progressive postpartum depression is widespread. This is not just an American problem. It is universal.

Deanne Tilton Durfee, executive director of the Los Angeles County Inter-Agency Task Force on Child Abuse and Neglect and chair of a panel composed of experts on child abuse states, "When it comes to deaths of infants and small children...at the hands of parents or caretakers, society has responded in a strangely muffled, seemingly disinterested way." She also asserts, "The parents commonly have a history of previous violence, social isolation, substance abuse, and poverty."

In one such case, for example, Suzanne Barnard, a social worker in the children's division of the American Humane Association, recalls meeting with a woman in Colorado who had killed her infant child, "She had substance abuse and mental illness problems. Her husband had left them. She felt that she had no future and that the child had no future. I asked if she knew about all the ways she could get help, from public assistance to family members. She had no idea. She had been abused herself. I felt profound sadness and helplessness. Although I had access to community resources, we hadn't connected in time to prevent this tragedy."

Among other major findings of the panel of experts on child abuse headed by Durfee:

❧ Head trauma is the leading cause of child abuse deaths. "Shaken baby syndrome" is so lethal that up to 25 percent of its victims die and most survivors suffer brain damage.

❧ Domestic violence is strongly linked to child abuse deaths. An estimated 50 percent of homes where adult violence occurs tend to also have child abuse or neglect.

❧ Many states lack adequate legal sanctions.

VERY YOUNG CHILDREN ARE particularly susceptible to fatal abuse. These victims are called the "invisible kids" because their age leaves them largely out of sight of the community. In a study of the Department of Justice, investigators reported that death of children for reason of murder usually followed a pattern of child abuse. In 80 percent of the cases, the parent who killed a child had also abused that child.

An example of this statistic is the case of Annie Marshall of Port Orange, Florida. Annie was 14 years old, 4'8" tall, and weighed 28 pounds when she died, curled in a fetal position in a corner of a room. Suffering from cerebral palsy, she was starved for three months prior to her death. On the morning of her death, Kathryn Allen, Annie's mother, fed Annie's two sisters breakfast, along with her 1-year-old son. Her boyfriend, Lawrence Kuzmovich, took the girls to school, then came home and dialed the non-emergency number at the police department.

Very often one child is chosen for abuse and eventual death by a parent. In this case the child was born with cerebral palsy and was not a "perfect" child, for which she apparently was punished.

Many researchers feel that the major message inherent in cases like the one cited above is to appreciate how important it is to educate people to help them become better parents. However, education on parenting alone is comparable to using a Band-Aid to stop a gushing wound from hemorrhaging. This speaks to the inability to recognize that there is major pathology present in these women and that medical intervention is paramount. In addition, education on parenting ought to include current, accurate information on PPD and PPPD so that expectant mothers can determine whether they are at risk.

THE MEDICAL VIEWPOINT

It is very difficult for women in the throes of progressive postpartum depression to identify the gravity of the problem. Professional or family intervention may be required just to recognize that there is a problem. Knowing in advance the statistics and who is at risk will give some common sense ideas to the public and to clinicians about how to deal with this problem.

While most popular books profess to cover everything "from conception to birth and beyond," closer examination reveals that the only references to serious mood swings after the birth of a child were attributed to problems related to "body image, diet, exercise, fatigue and care of the baby." None of these publications mentions medical or hormonal implications.

In perusing these books, I have found only nondescript references to mood swings during the postpartum period in which new mothers who feel angry or depressed are simply directed to talk to their doctor about it and are told that these symptoms should subside after a few weeks. Well, what if these feelings continue? Without an official declaration that all these symptoms and more are distinct possibilities for the "at risk" woman, a woman is not in a position to know 1) whether she is at risk and 2) that if she is, she is particularly susceptible to a prolonged and possibly tragic course of depression.

At long last, the fourth edition of *The Diagnostic and Statistical Manual of Mental Disorders*, published in 1994, and commonly called DSM-IV by clinicians, now gives some information on PPD to the medical professions. Called a "Postpartum Onset Specifier," PPD is listed under the heading "Mood Disorders."[19]

Unfortunately, this means that postpartum depression is not yet designated as a distinct disorder. *The Manual* does not differentiate the "postpartum onset specifier" as an entity unto itself, but rather a specifier to be applied to the current or most recent major depressive, manic, or mixed episode in major depressive disorder; bipolar I disorder; bipolar II disorder; or to brief psychotic disorder illnesses. Most of these conditions are in the category of mood disorders. They are serious conditions, resulting in behavior very often beyond the patient's control. Usually they are familial (genetically predisposed) much as postpartum depression. In addition they are treatable once the correct diagnosis is made, just as postpartum depression is.

The Manual describes the onset as being within four weeks after delivery of a child, and that a fluctuating course of mood lability may be more common in postpartum episodes than in any other mood disorder. Suicidal ideation, obsessional thoughts regarding violence to the child, lack of concentration, and agitation can be additional manifestations. *The Manual* also discusses delusions which could accompany the depression (e.g., the newborn is possessed by the devil, has special powers, or is destined for a terrible fate).

While infanticide can occur in severe postpartum mood episodes without specific delusions or hallucinations, it is most often associated with postpartum psychotic episodes characterized by command hallucinations to kill the infant or delusions that the infant is possessed. Postpartum mood (major depressive, manic, or mixed) episodes with psychotic features appear to occur in from 1 in 500 to 1 in 1000 deliveries and may be more common in postpartum women.

To cite an example, one victim of her mother's delusional symptoms was Tavielle Kiga, a five-year-old girl in Maine, who allegedly was starved to death by her mother. When her body was discovered, the state medical examiner said she died for lack of food and water. The girl's mother Tonia, 28, was charged with murder, after stating that she withheld food and water because the child was evil.

Another similar example of such an episode is the case of Judy Lynn Hessler, who stabbed her nine-month-old daughter, Rachel, 12 times, killing her in the process. In the days before the stabbing, Hessler stated she heard Rachel's voice saying, "Die, die." Hessler began to believe that Rachel wanted to die, so she would not have to have a life like her mother's.

Hessler had had a troubled life which included sexual abuse by members of her family and drug use. The attorney stated in court that Hessler was psychotic. The prosecution stated that being psychotic at the time of the murder did not establish the legal requirement to be found not guilty by reason of mental illness.

The risk of postpartum episodes with psychotic features is particularly increased for women with a prior history of postpartum mood episodes. It is also elevated for those with a prior history of any type of mood disorder. Once a woman has had a postpartum episode with psychotic features, the risk of recurrence with each subsequent delivery is between 30 percent and 50 percent. There is also some evidence of increased risk of postpartum psychotic episodes among women *without* a *personal history* of mood disorders, but *with* a *family history* of bipolar disorders (also known as manic-depressive illness).

Although I share this information with you, the reader, remember that these writings, descriptions and specifiers are written specifically for clinicians, who are diagnosing and treating. They are not written for the education of the general public. You could call this an example of "preaching to the choir." My opinion is that it is critical for the expectant mother, particularly one who is at risk for PPD or PPPD to understand the implications of this illness, for she will be the one most affected by diagnosis and her subsequent treatment.

In view of these statistics and cases, it is hard to understand why this subject is still so widely ignored by the medical profession and, subsequently, the general public. Why are there no books written for the general public addressing the problem right on the very same shelves with all the other books about "what the expectant mother should know"? What is the big secret the medical profession is keeping from women? Do they fear that women would not want to become pregnant?

Needless to say nothing would be further from the truth. If, in fact, women who had a history of depression or who were at risk because of family history could be properly counseled, they would be far more able to weather a pregnancy and birth. While information alone is no substitution for the medical treatment needed in some cases, education about PPD and PPPD is the first line of defense for all expectant mothers and their families when entering a new and life-changing experience.

3 | THE MEDICAL DISREGARD OF POSTPARTUM DEPRESSION

In trying to understand the complex picture of PPD, we have first to overcome years, if not centuries, of misinformation, negligence, and psychological dumping on women of what is now obviously a biochemically induced syndrome (or syndromes because there is more than one manifestation of PPD). But you will still find doctors, psychiatrists, and scientists arguing over the relative importance of the biochemical or psychogenic makeup of the emotional condition the new mother finds herself in.—Carol Dix in *The New Mother Syndrome: Coping with Postpartum Stress and Depression*[20]

OVER A DECADE AGO in 1985, medical journalist and author Carol Dix wrote a book called *The New Mother Syndrome*. It was an excellent description of postpartum depression (PPD) and it also contained a list of resources available to new mothers who recognize that they suffer from this disorder. In order to publicize her book, Ms. Dix appeared on numerous telelvision shows, including *Donahue* and *The Oprah Winfrey Show.* More than 12 years after that national media exposure, society and the medical establishment still do little to educate women about this easily recognizable syndrome.

To reinforce this, we have seen a rash of sensational cases of child abuse and murder cases, which have recently received a great deal of attention. Now, thanks to these horror stories, will the medical community and the general public finally begin to take notice of this very common illness?

Remember Ariel's story from Chapter One? Why did the obstetrician miss the early signs of a mood disorder? The simplest answer is that medical students and residents in medicine do not learn about postpartum depression in medical school. If they do, the condition is usually downplayed as a transient condition. Despite the findings on PPD cited in the 1994 DSM-IV, described in the previous chapter, the connection between postpartum depression and mood disorders has not yet been widely accepted by clinicians and consequently has not been widely publicized. The information falls between the cracks, somewhere between psychiatry, psychology, and obstetrics.

Historically, there has been a serious gap in communication among professionals regarding this subject. Part of the problem is that the symptoms are so varied that many illnesses may be suspected. Not only are the symptoms varied, but each cultural and ethnic group typically expresses the symptoms according to their own background, country of origin, and religion so that diagnosing correctly can involve not only a clear understanding of pathology, but also of the cultural differences in expressing it.

From the 1800s until the 1950s, most of the writings regarding postpartum behavior was observational from the perspective of the researchers and clinicians. It was not until 1952 that there was even any effort to find a proper nomenclature for the disorder.

Even today, clinicians are slow and sometimes reluctant to treat the symptoms of postpartum depression as a medical illness requiring medical treatment. I feel it is important to stress that although *most* psychiatrists and psychologists may be equipped to diagnose and recommend treatment, a dangerous gap in the knowledge of other medical disciplines still remains.

This gap largely involves the obstetrician, gynecologist, pediatrician, family doctor, and internists. And these clinicians are the only ones the mothers and their partners, family, and friends have to rely on for guidance and diagnosis during the months before and after the birth of a child. They are in the position to be on the front lines of defense for the uuninformed.

Dr. Veronika Solt of Columbia-Presbyterian Medical Center stresses that a closer liaison between obstetricians, gynecologists, and psychiatrists is necessary to promote evaluation, counseling, and recognition for women who are unaware, negligent, or have no family support to insist on treatment. I agree, but I also believe that this essential liaison will not happen until each specialty of medicine teaches the importance of recognizing and treating depression in women.

Other physicians echo my sentiment. According to Dr. Michael O'Hara, professor and chair of the Department of Psychology at the University of Iowa, primary care physicians could play a much larger role than they presently do in identifying women with postpartum depression or those who are at risk of developing it. These physicians should also be able to direct the woman toward proper medical treatment. "They should be alert, implement low level screening procedures for depression, and certainly give women the opportunity to talk about their feelings," O'Hara says.

As it stands now, clinicians tend to send the patient to marital counseling, parent effectiveness training, and other forms of support groups, simply because historically, postpartum depression has not been seen as a serious medical illness. Many still consider its manifestations to be normal, to simply be the "baby blues." Therefore, they fail to identify an illness in time to prevent its sometimes inevitable progression.

The real answer to this professional dilemma, of course, is in the teaching and training of all these medical and clinical people. They *are* in a position to warn, watch, help, and control the manifestations of this uninvited guest—depression—to the new mother's home.

New books and broader media coverage are finally disseminating information that gives expectant mothers themselves, and/or those who care about them, greater power to recognize their own condition. This emergence of an informed public will also help to diminish the resistance of professionals.

Even doctors who recognize the importance of educating expectant mothers, their families, spouses, and friends, have typically not seen discussion of postpartum depression as part of their role. Likewise many psychiatrists, psychologists, and other health clinicians who do not have the necessary information, fail to inform their patients. Therefore the general public remains uninformed. If all these professionals are not in the business of preventative medical care, whose job should it be? Similarly, I believe that professionals are responsible for a better informed public because they are in the best position to have access to the most recent medical data on postpartum depression. New findings on the help now available to mothers at risk have been distributed almost exclusively in professional medical journals and forums geared to the clinician—not the lay public.

In fact the task of informing their patients about this issue should be the job of all these professionals because postpartum depression *is* a medical illness that affects the child as well as the mother. As Dr. O'Hara states: "If untreated, a mother's depression can compromise the development of the child."

The effect on the child is another compelling reason to urge prevention and early treatment of postpartum treatment—a double toll—on the infant as well as the mother.

Only recently have clinicians begun to explore and identify the high-risk expectant mother. Symptoms during pregnancy would, of course, be a compelling sign of the probability of an impending postpartum depression. But usually there are no signs prior to the birth.

Insufficient emphasis has also been given to genetic predisposition. This could be easily addressed in a complete family history which could be taken routinely in the obstetrician's office. Additionally, information regarding stresses in the pregnant mother's life should be gathered as part of this survey. These stresses could include financial strain, marital problems, responsibility of other children, work pressures or any problematic relationships.

I reiterate Dr. O'Hara's assertion that primary care physicians could play a far more important role in identifying women who may be at risk. The good doctor, right on point, also emphasizes the importance of screening procedures.

My point is that if professionals remain unconcerned and uncommunicative, how then can mothers feel secure?

❤ ❤ ❤

WHEN I QUESTIONED a number of colleagues regarding *The Diagnostic Manual*, many said they believed that postpartum depression was not included in it. This is alarming, and certainly bad news for expectant mothers, for if the bulk of clinicians did not expect to find these indicators, then how can the general public expect to be informed?

Those clinicians who do have a knowledge of the DSM-IV and what it contains can read that many women feel especially guilty about having depressive feelings at a time when they believe they should be happy. They may be reluctant to discuss their symptoms or their negative feeling toward the child. Less-than-optimal development of the mother-infant relationship may result from the clinical condition itself or from separations from the infant.

This information is readily available to anyone in the health care field. I personally was impressed by the inclusion of this clear-cut description in the well-known manual by which all psychiatric diagnosis is included. Now it becomes our mission to educate professionals as well as the general public.

I recently experienced a first-hand example of this problem of ignorance in the medical community while chatting with a gynecologist friend of mine. I have sent many patients to this doctor over the years and always held him in the highest regard. I told him the topic of my upcoming book was postpartum depression. He stunned me with his response: "Not much of that going around these days. Most women usually resolve their 'psychological' issues during prenatal care," he said.

"What about their hormonal responses?" I asked. He had no answer.

My doctor friend and I parted without any resolution. He remained convinced that postpartum depression is all a psychological issue. His attitude is difficult for me to accept. For over forty years, the evidence that mood disorders have a physiological and biochemical basis has continued to accumulate, verified by a mountain of research and documentation. I can hardly believe that respected and seemingly progressive physicians can be so antiquated in their thinking, a sign of how widespread this thinking remains within the health care professions.

It would behoove clinicians in general to look at the well accepted anthropological views of the rituals surrounding the postpartum period as a cue toward what we may be overlooking in our own culture. An outstanding book, entitled *Postpartum Psychiatric Illness: A Picture Puzzle*,[21] contains a collection of writings by many clinicians from all over the world on this subject. Albeit a brilliant anthology, it is not on the shelves of popular books for the public, and is most likely only easily accessible to professionals.

One chapter by Lawrence Dean Kruckman entitled "An Anthropological View of Postpartum Depression" illustrates viewpoints from China, Nepal, Spain, Guatemala, the Caribbean, the Philippines, Nigeria, Kenya, Mexico, and India. In China and Kenya, for example, close support and care are provided by the husband, parents, and relatives. Therefore, postpartum depression is uncommon (or goes unreported).[22] Guatemalans, for example, believe it is important to keep the mother warm and maintain a regime of confinement. Mexicans use a special diet, advise heat treatment, and use elaborate medications. In Punjab, India, seclusion for five days is expected, except for female relatives and the midwife.

Yucatan relatives come to greet the new baby only after the eight-day seclusion of mother and baby. Among the Ibos of Nigeria, the new mother and infant are secluded in the "fattening room," a special hut in the family compound. They are cared for by older women. The new mother's only functions are to eat, sleep, and care for her baby.[23]

In addition to restrictions on a woman's physical activities, some cultures and religions regard the postpartum period as a time of impurity. The recuperative period in some groups revolves around the care by female relatives of the new mother.[24] There are rules regarding rest, regaining strength, and special care for the baby and mother. Some countries practice forty days of religious observances, while others call for an eight-day period.

Other societies may take the behaviors and reactions of a new mother into consideration, and deal with them as expected. They build policy, structure, and rituals around the birth. Therefore, it is clear, that despite the differences in the perspectives of various societies, cultures, countries, and religions, one significant fact stands out: most cultures acknowledge the necessity for some type of elaborate social, biological, or religious ritual following birth and during the postpartum period.

By contrast, we in America expect the mother to leave the hospital within 24 hours to two days, arrive home, be happy and joyful, take care of home and family, tend the new baby, and get back to work within the time allotted for maternity leave. I call these "drive-by births." To me this does not imply common sense, nor is it a very "civilized" approach for a so-called modern culture.

The medical viewpoint in the U.S. is that postpartum depression operates in a kind of bubble or vacuum, as a somewhat normal entity unto itself. We are generally bereft of the cultural rituals that support a woman through the postpartum period. We do not view the perinatal period as a time when possible serious depression may occur and have a negative, long-lasting effect on the mother and the child.

One of the difficulties for the new mother in seeking and/or getting help from a health care professional is that despite much literature describing these symptoms as a major mental disorder, there is little concurrence among psychiatrists about the nature—or even the existence—of postpartum illness.

Dr. James Alexander Hamilton, who has written extensively on the subject of postpartum depression, maintains that sometimes when symptoms diminish, or become less apparent, women are able to conceal and suppress the behavior—at least for a time. However, he contends, episodes of hallucinations and delusions may persist and recur unpredictably. This certainly explains another obstacle in diagnosis.

This controversy over the precise nature of PPD also arises in a re-examination of the Sudden Infant Death Syndrome (SIDS) deaths. Researchers and police are now looking for signs that the babies once thought to be victims of SIDS were, rather, victims of child abuse and filicide. In 1997, the publication of the book *The Death of the Innocents* by Richard Firstman and Jamie Talan, prompted police to re-examine a number of deaths that had been attributed to SIDS. The authors cite a 1972 study which led many to believe that SIDS ran in families. The authors claim that about one-third of the 155 babies treated in Massachusetts General Hospital for repeated episodes of SIDS between 1972 and 1975 could have been abused. While no one is asserting that vast numbers of babies believed to have died of SIDS actually were killed by their parents, some might have been, say these experts.

In one family particularly, the mother was discovered to have killed all five of her children. Waneta Hoyt, age 49, was convicted of murder and was given the minimum sentence of 15 years to life for each of the five counts.

At the time of the deaths, doctors suspected Sudden Infant Death Syndrome (SIDS). Last year, however, Hoyt confessed that from 1965 to 1971, she smothered Erik, Julie, Molly, and Noah Hoyt to stop them from crying. None of the children was older than 27 months.

The case was reopened in 1992 when a prosecutor became suspicious after reading a medical journal account of the deaths.

I'm sure that there are a percentage of *real* SIDS deaths. At the same time, it is likely that a substantial number of mothers have suffocated their babies when depressed. More scrutiny will have to be exercised in order to make a true determination.

However, despite the fact that PPD is often either misdiagnosed or simply not recognized at all, as Dr. Daniel Maier-Katkin points out in an article called "Mothers Who Kill" in the *Miami Herald*,[26] according to a 1987 study done in Scotland, the likelihood of a woman of childbearing age being admitted to a psychiatric hospital with a diagnosis of psychosis was 22 times greater during the month after giving birth than at any other time.

Despite scientific studies like this one that add to the evidence of PPD as a common condition with potentially horrific repercussions when untreated, making real progress can be frustratingly slow. A November 2, 1997 article in *The New York Times Magazine* by Steven Pinker called "Why They Kill Their Newborns" was quite shocking to me in its ignorance and blatant misinformation. The subtitle read, "A mother who murders her baby commits an immoral act, but not necessarily a pathological one. Neonaticide may be a product of 'maternal wiring.'" This opinion flies in the face of all that we have learned regarding the human behavior of mothers and their children. And more importantly, it does nothing to solve the problem.[26]

Martin Daly and Margo Wilson, both psychologists, argue in this article that humans have the capacity to kill our newborns and that it is built into the biological design of our parental emotions. This anthropological viewpoint may hold when examining very early human evolutionary history, as these psychologists have. When humans were still hunter-gatherers, babies had only a small chance of survival to adulthood. In such societies, they explain, "a woman lets a newborn die when its prospects for survival to adulthood are poor. The forecast might be based on abnormal signs in the infant, or on bad circumstances for successful motherhood at the time—she might be burdened with older children, beset by war or famine or without a husband or social support."

If these two psychologists hold to the idea that as a modern society, we are still in the throes of the forces shaping our early ancestors, when 'survival of the fittest' was the order of the day, then they must refute evolution and bonding. Daly and Wilson attempt to make a case that neonaticide is not an illness, but part of our culture. As a scientist of modern-day human behavior, I must disagree. The days of the hunter-gatherers have long since past and societal standards and moral codes have changed through the ages. If we are to believe that humans have evolved and that we measure behavior by modern day society's standards, then I must disagree that anyone would commit an act that is: 1) criminal and 2) immoral as a result of "maternal wiring."

Daly and Wilson do assert that once a mother bonds with her newborn (presumably after the immediate postpartum "triage"), she is imprinted with a lifelong attachment to the baby. Why would any woman who has previously never displayed criminal or immoral behavior commit such a ego-dystonic act? Surely she must be distraught and possibly cognitively impaired beyond reason.

The cases of teenage girls murdering their infants may come under another category of depression, a reactive one, stemming not only from the hormonal activity, but also from fear of society, family, and their own perception of an inability to care for the child.

Despite the difficulties in determining a definitive model for postpartum depression, the one thing doctors and patients alike can and should agree upon (based on statistics and current studies) is that postpartum depression is not the rarity most people would like to believe. It is only when the doctors who currently belittle postpartum depression and progressive postpartum depression as a passing, self-indulgent phase of new motherhood recognize these conditions as mental illnesses, that lives will be saved.

My point in relating these discrepancies among medical professionals regarding the nature of PPD is not to argue the point about how complicated the diagnostic process is. In fact, my point is exactly the opposite. Since there is so much literature describing the symptoms of postpartum depression as part of a major medical disorder, I believe that if professionals commonly acknowledged postpartum depression as an entity, the diagnosis would be altogether simplified. Clinicians then would look at postpartum depression as a possible *first* diagnosis.

4 | TREATMENT

Despite our ability to treat the [manic-depressive] illness, patients and their physicians often either fail to recognize it or are reluctant to acknowledge it. Consequently, not even one in three receives treatment.—Frederick K. Goodwin and Kay Redfield Jamison in Introduction of *Manic-Depressive Illness*[27]

ACCURATE DIAGNOSIS AND proper treatment are inseparable. To define postpartum depression as "OB Blues" or "baby blues" even when the condition becomes severe and long lived, trivializes what is, in fact, a serious and debilitating illness that strikes only women. I contend that no psychotherapy or behavior modification in the world will stop a real postpartum depression. They can only delay it, perhaps only to reappear at a future date—ergo, *progressive* postpartum depression. The real issue for readers and the most important service of this book concerns this question: Is there a remedy for postpartum depression and for progressive postpartum depression?

Mood disorders, including postpartum depression and progressive postpartum depression, can be effectively treated today with modern medicine. When left untreated, they can become progressive and perpetuate from generation to generation. That is not to say that the genetic predisposition disappears if the condition is treated. With treatment, however, as in any other genetic illness, mood disorders can be controlled and are no longer a threat to well-being.

THE EFFECT OF POSTPARTUM DEPRESSION ON THE INFANT

The November 1996 *Clinical Psychiatry News* published this front page headline: "Treat Postpartum Depression Early." Written by Carl Sherman, a contributing editor, the article warned psychiatrists of the dangers of this illness.[28] Though there have been references to postpartum issues in the past, this was the first front-page PPD story to appear in a professional context.

In the article, Michael O'Hara, Ph.D., a professor and chair of psychology at the University of Iowa, urged prevention and early treatment to avoid the double toll—on the infant as well as the mother. Clinicians, now, are beginning to explore and identify the high risk expectant mother and the effect on the new baby. My desire to emphasize treatment lies in the fact that postpartum depression takes this double toll. Dr. O'Hara stipulates how: "If untreated, depression can compromise the development of the child and is likely to recur." The new statistics show prevalence of postpartum depression in 13 percent of births, according to an analysis of 59 studies conducted by Dr. O'Hara and Annette M. Swain.

"We know that the impact of a postpartum depression on the early mother-child relationship is negative and substantial," says Dr. Lynn Grush, associate director of the perinatal psychiatric clinical research program at Massachusetts General Hospital in Boston. In addition, Dr. Grush points out that not only is the relationship between mother and child impaired, but the negative interaction affects the child's development, as well as the child's cognition.

Dr. Veronika Solt of Columbia-Presbyterian Medical Center in New York City conducted a recent study of 71 inner-city women which reinforces Dr. Grush's findings. Dr. Solt found that depressed women were significantly less likely to breast-feed than others. The depression evidently affected the bonding and reflected an overall lack of interest in and physical contact with the baby.

According to a September 1997 issue of *The Harvard Mental Health Letter* (a publication from Harvard Medical School), a mother's disturbed emotions cause distorted thinking and often become centered on confusing thoughts about her baby. In truth, the depression has twisted her thinking. This is known as cognitive deficit. In turn, because of her self-engrossed state, the mother is perhaps unable to be responsive to the baby's needs, or her moods may be so changeable that the baby may mirror her emotions. The article goes on to describe the distinct differences between the responses of a child of a depressed mother as compared to the responses of the child of a mother not suffering from depression.

In the article's description of mother's dynamics, her depressed state and her concerns about her child make her "silent, irritable, inattentive, lacking in playfulness, and unresponsive to the child's need. Infants are sensitive to the moods of their parents from birth. At three months, children of depressed mothers smile less than average, turn their heads away from adults, and seem more upset when they look at their mother's face than when she leaves the room. The failure to establish an emotional tie with the mother may have long-term effects as well."[20]

Similarly, at an annual meeting in Toronto of the American Academy of Child and Adolescent Psychiatry, Phyllis Zelkowitz, Ed.D., reported that "the mother's dysfunction appeared to have an impact on infant development. In particular, motor development was negatively correlated with maternal anxiety."[30]

POSTPARTUM DEPRESSION
AND MOOD DISORDERS

Clinical research clearly shows that illnesses associated with pregnancy and the postpartum period have long divided clinicians. Even such ancient physicians as Hippocrates, Celsus, and Galen, felt that pregnancy had a role in the precipitation of bizarre behavior.

I have, in previous chapters, addresses the issues of: 1) hormonal changes; 2) altered body image; 3) conflicts relating to pregnancy; and 4) the dynamics of assuming motherhood. Even though these topics are commonly accepted as evidence of the changes a woman undergoes during her childbearing years, controversy continues to surround the opinions of *how* these changes affect the new mother, her baby, and the family.

Dr. Deborah A. Sichel, Clinical Associate at the Perinatal Psychiatry Clinical Research Program at Massachusetts General Hospital in Boston, and instructor in psychiatry at Harvard Medical School reports: "New information suggests that the postpartum period is one of substantial vulnerability, especially with respect to worsening of preexisting psychiatric disorders."

This would include unipolar* depression, bipolar disorder, anxiety disorders, all mood or affective disorders. Her work concerning anxiety disorders during pregnancy and the postpartum period demonstrates how quickly and how severely ill patients can become in the early postpartum period.

With respect to affective (mood) disorders, further research is required to distinguish early from later postpartum syndromes. The most recent work suggests "that a subgroup of patients are more vul-

---

*Definition: a single-gene trait; e.g. as in having only depression, and not mania.

nerable to early postpartum illness—patients who are affectively well at delivery and become severely symptomatic within two weeks.

"If some of these patients prove to be identifiable before the onset of illness, we may be able to prevent or mitigate their symptoms by early pharmacotherapeutic, hormonal, and/or psychotherapeutic interventions. We are interested in the neuropharmacologic mechanisms by which the 'estrogen withdrawal state' of the postpartum period may accelerate the onset of illness."[31]

OBSESSIVE COMPULSIVE DISORDER AND CONCOMITANT DISORDERS IN POSTPARTUM DEPRESSION

In 1993, Drs. Sichel, Cohen, Simmock, and Rosenbaum[32] conducted a study with fifteen women displaying obsessive compulsive symptoms, new to them and having begun at the postpartum period, who were evaluated by reviewing their treatment records. They clearly met the criteria in *The Diagnostic Manual.* The results showed that these women had a set of symptoms which were comprised of disabling, intrusive, and obsessional thoughts to harm their babies. In reality, they had not harmed their respective babies, but it was clear that clinicians caring for women postpartum should have been aware of the impact of these symptoms on the mother as well as on the child's well-being.

A very interesting and somewhat atypical case that illustrates the importance of recognizing these symptoms postpartum is that of a woman who on the surface appeared to be the "perfect mother." This young mother was super-conscientious about taking care of her new baby. She diapered him numerous times, always cleaning his skin with all the necessary applications. She became increasingly fearful about not keeping her baby clean enough. At the same time, she washed her hands excessively, afraid to carry germs to her baby. This continued until a family member noticed that the baby's skin was rubbed raw from over-cleaning. The pediatrician had thought that this mother was a "perfect mother" and that the baby's increasingly reddened skin was just a serious diaper rash.

When symptoms are presented in a new mother, the clinician must first make certain that there is no physical cause, such as a thyroid condition (common during and after pregnancy). Because of its clinical similarity to postpartum depression, hypothyroidism should always be considered. Hashimoto's syndrome, one type of a thyroid involvement, is not uncommon following a pregnancy and is frequently associated with a depressive state. Therefore thyroid studies should be an important component in developing a diagnosis of postpartum depression or progressive postpartum depression.

BIOCHEMICAL TREATMENT AND MEDICATIONS

Numerous forms of treatment have developed in the last 40 years. Today many medications such as lithium, anti-convulsives, anti-depressants, and other mood stabilizers enable patients suffering from many categories of mood disorders to lead satisfying and productive lives without chronic suffering.

Progressive postpartum depression can be identified in its early and less dangerous stages. And once PPPD has been diagnosed, we are armed with medical and psychotherapeutic treatments which can counteract the effects of this potentially dangerous illness. Speedy recognition by family, friends, and doctors can allow the woman to be diagnosed and treated immediately, before the situation becomes chronic. A mother who is diagnosed early in her illness need not travel down the path that leads to madness. She can be as productive as she was before the onset of the illness.

One of my patients who suffered a serious postpartum depression after the birth of her first child opted to begin treatment immediately after the births of her subsequent four healthy and happy children. Another patient, who had early depressions and mood instability, began treatment during the pregnancy, and subsequently has a bouncing healthy boy.

PROPHYLACTIC TREATMENT

Just there are a number of reasons to treat PPD, there are a number of alternatives in treatment. For example, a woman at risk (one with a history of depression) might consider prophylactic medication close to the time of delivery or directly after delivery.

A great deal of literature now in medical journals and books recommends prophylactic treatment with medications for women who have had a previous postpartum episode or for women who have a history of bipolar disorder (Ayd, 1991; Van Gent, 1993; McKenzie and Deakin, 1993; and Cohen, Sichel, Robertson, Heckscher, and Rosenbaum, 1995).

At an update on psychopharmacology sponsored by New York University Post-Graduate Medical School, Dr. Barbara Parry of the School of Medicine at the University of California, San Diego stated, "Women with a history of postpartum depression are at high risk of recurrence and may benefit from prophylactic pharmacotherapy shortly after delivery." She reported that although the incidence of psychiatric disorders drops substantially during pregnancy, the first month postpartum brings a steep rise in risk that can persist for months.

Like Dr. Parry, I advocate preventative treatment for those who have had previous postpartum episodes. Dr. Parry's observations and research are in concurrence with my experiences in that preventative treatment averts future tragedy. In one series of patients with histories of mood disorders, continued recurrent depressions were seen in more than 60 percent of the untreated, but only 4.3 percent (1 of 23) in those who were treated after delivery. Dr. Parry stated that medication can be initiated within twelve hours after delivery.

One interesting case described in a psychiatry textbook is of a 33-year-old woman with a history of three prior pregnancies. All the prior pregnancies had been accompanied by hypo-manic episodes requiring hospitalization for three to four weeks. She had never been sick, except in association with pregnancy. There was no history in the family for affective disorder. She had been referred for evaluation for medication therapy.

She was a contented housewife and mother with three healthy children, a marriage without major problems, and a healthy sexual adjustment. At the fourth birth, a mood stabilizer was administered immediately after delivery, and no hypo-manic behavior recurred. Medication was discontinued at three months postpartum without onset of illness.[33]

Fortunately, we are now in a time in which there are many new and effective medications on the market. Treatment for depression is no longer in the "shotgun" era, in which doctors had very few choices to control symptoms and tried one thing or another until something finally worked.

Just as there are a variety of symptoms involved in depressions— dysthymia, obsessive-compulsions, anxiety, panic, paranoia, delusions, and hallucinations—so are there as many medications for treating them.

In the past there were only antidepressants called tricyclics (called TCAs) on the market, in use since 1958. The tricyclic group included the following drugs: Tofranil (imipramine); Elavil (amitriptyline); Norpramin (desipramine); Pamelor (nortriptyline);

Vivactil (protriptyline); Anafranil (clomipramine), also recommended for obsessive-compulsive symptoms; and Surmontil (trimipramine). Some related medications called tetracyclics are Ludiomil (maprotiline) and Asendin (amoxapine).

A second group of antidepressant medications are the MAOIs, an acronym for Monoamine Oxidase Inhibitors. These were successfully used in Europe for many years before being tested in the United States and have dietary restrictions for users. They include: Marplan (isocarboxazid); Nardil (phenelzine); and Parnate (tranylcypromine).

These original medications have been used successfully for depression for the past thirty years. However, while these medications helped many people, they also had side effects which gave more resistant patients an excuse to stop taking them. Therefore compliance was always a difficult part of the treatment. Furthermore since there were always some who did not respond to TCAs or MAOIs, or couldn't tolerate the side effects, a new group arrived on the market called SSRIs, an acronym for Selective Serotonin Reuptake Inhibitors. These were shown to have minimal side effects when compared to the older variety of tricyclics. Although some patients who could not tolerate the side effects have been changed to the newer medications by their doctors, I hasten to add that many people are still taking one of the original drugs and continue to be helped.

The SSRIs included Prozac (fluoxetine); Zoloft (sertraline); Paxil (paroxetine); Luvox (fluvoxamine), another medication recommended for obsessive symptoms; and Serzone (nefazadone). A separate group in increased use are Wellbutrin (buporprion) and Effexor (venlafaxine). Still being used also is Deseryl (trazodone).

Major tranquilizers like Thorazine (chlorpromazine), Mellaril (thioridazine), Trilafon (perphenazine), Stelazine (trifluoperazine), Haldol (haloperidol), Loxapine (loxapine), Navane (thiothixene),

Clozaril (clozapine), Risperdal (risperidone), and Serentil (mesoridazine) are still in use for severe symptoms and quick relief. But because of the side effects, and the more effective ways of treating the underlying mood disorder, they are being used only when other medications have not been effective.

There are newer and even more effective medications to have appeared on the market recently in the category of minor tranquilizers: Xanax (alprazolam); Ativan (lorazepam); and Klonopin (clonazepam). These are all habit-forming, as is Valium (diazepam), and thus, are best prescribed only on a short-term basis. A newer, non-habit-forming tranquilizer called Buspar (buspirone) is now on the market as well.

Mood stabilizers are the miracle medications for cycling (highs and lows) and for long-term therapy, which for many people go hand in hand with mood disorders. They include: Eskalith or Lithonate (lithium carbonate); Tegretol (carbamazepine); and Depakote or Depakene (valporic acid). These stabilizers help to stabilize the metabolism and also to enhance the efficacy of the antidepressants. More recently some doctors are using thyroid hormones such as Cytomel, to boost the antidepressant's action. Lithium especially has been a boon to thousands. Recently the anticonvulsants such as Tegretol and Depakote are being used increasingly.

It is important to note that doctors are recommending that many of their patients stay on medications indefinitely. There is no reason to think that with recovery or even marked improvement the medications should be discontinued. In fact, it would be foolhardy, since improvement is an obvious result of the medications. It is essential to understand that stabilizers such as Lithium, Depakote, and Tegretol may be necessary for lifetime stabilization medications for mood disorders. They serve not only as a control for symptoms, but more importantly perhaps, as a prophylactic against future episodes.

My intention in describing these drugs groups here is not to promote any one group in particular—each group has its pros and cons—but rather to relate the numerous medication options that are now available to people suffering from depression and/or mood disorders. However, despite the wide array of potential treatments, it is still essential for anyone considering prophylactic treatment to proceed with caution. Consultations with appropriate medical professionals to determine the treatment that best suits the individual needs of each patient are absolutely vital. And in all cases, all medications must be prescribed by a competent medical doctor, preferably a psychopharmacologist, specializing in mood disorders. This is important for rapid recovery and to prevent harmful interactions between medications. Only a physician conversant with the literature of the newest medications and the patient's physical condition would be appropriate to prescribe a safe and efficient regimen.

Similarly, I would be remiss if I did not inform you that psychotherapy and education regarding the illness and the treatment are essential to recovering and staying well. Various types of psychotherapy have been particularly helpful. I personally have seen excellent results with individual therapy, using cognitive therapy as a model. Group therapy has been extremely helpful to women in recognizing that they are not alone in the frightening world of postpartum depression.

SUPPORT GROUPS, EDUCATIONAL COUNSELING, AND PSYCHOTHERAPY

If women have symptoms from the stresses involved with postpartum, such as lack of support, negative life events, or other pressures, there are many interventions. One is group therapy, suggested during pregnancy, which at the very least offers insight to the incidence of depression and also serves as a support system.

Dr. Michael O'Hara, professor and chair of the Department of Psychology at the University of Iowa, is presently conducting a study exploring whether interpersonal therapy can help prevent postpartum depression in women at risk, but results are not available yet. Other studies show that psychotherapy as well as medical treatment is indicated after the acute phase of the illness is past. This therapy is usually directed at the conflict areas that have become evident during this very difficult period.

A study of young mothers who feared that they might murder their children found that the thought itself is a sign of approaching insanity. Sixteen mothers with this clinical picture were evaluated in interviews. Seven of them entered psychotherapy and improved. The prognosis of these women who have had systematic psychotherapy is good (Chapman, Chapman-Santana, and Teixeira, 1996).[34]

Even when psychotherapy was not possible, as was the case in nine of the women in the study cited above, they were strongly reassured and explanations were given about the nature of their problem. This encouragement and clarification helped them improve significantly.

Support groups and educational counseling have also proven to be valuable, especially during the pregnancy.

FAMILY AND FRIENDS

Mobilizing personal, emotional support systems is an important adjunct to either medical treatment or psychotherapy or both. Here lies the importance of education of family, friends, and partners. My hope is that this and other information will be read by mothers and expectant mothers, or those who care about them, bypassing the resistance the professionals have displayed regarding this tragic illness.

WHO CAN HELP?
THE CHAIN OF RECOGNITION

The obstetrician could be the first person to recognize the symptoms of postpartum depression. A postpartum clinical depression is not "natural" or "normal," no matter what anyone might tell a suffering new mother, says Dr. Mark Gold in *The Good News About Depression.* He quotes Dr. David Danforth, professor emeritus of obstetrics and gynecology at Northwestern University School of Medicine in Chicago: "Most obstetricians don't have great insight into the emotional problems of childbirth."[35]

It is widely accepted by knowledgeable clinicians that the "at risk" group of women can develop very severe affective symptoms, symptoms of mood instability, rapidly following delivery. Certainly by being able to identify the vulnerable woman, we could prevent problems by early intervention.

This intervention could occur after a doctor takes a careful and systematic history during the first visit. This history should include the expectant mother's and her family's background. This detailed questioning process should reveal the presence of any characteristics in the family that have been associated with a positive history of mood disorders. These may include but aren't limited to the following traits:

➤ addictions (alcohol and/or drugs);
➤ early truancy at school age;
➤ oppositional behavior;
➤ hyper-sexual behavior;
➤ sociopathy;
➤ multiple marriages;
➤ multiple job history;

❥ "ups and downs" in business;

❥ color blindness (males in the family);

❥ bouts of depression, suicidal ideation, violent acting out, and grandiosity;

❥ suicide.

At least two characteristics should be apparent to identify the mother at risk.

Dr. O'Hara reports "that virtually any stressor occurring in a woman's life at around the time of the birth of a baby increases her risk of postpartum illness, particularly affective illness."[36]

The pediatrician or an emergency room doctor are typically trained to focus on only the baby and not the mother, even though symptoms may be evident in her and her alone. The mother may have become unkempt, while baby is dressed to a tee, or the mother may have become hyper-sexual in a way that was not common for her previously.

Many doctors who are accustomed to dealing with new mothers often take for granted that all the mother's questions and complaints are simply the result of her insecurity and/or fatigue. Terming them hysteria, they frequently ignore them. These doctors are second in line of importance of being able to listen carefully, ask the right questions, and have the right answers to be of immediate assistance to the family, refer to the proper clinician, and thereby have a very important role in saving the mother and child from possible disaster.

This clinician may be the *only* one to hear of the emerging symptoms of the mother at risk. The practitioner and assistants, if unable to hear or pick up the clues from mothers' descriptions of problems, can carefully scrutinize the condition of the child:

❥ Are there signs of malnutrition—either through nursing or bottle-feeding?

❥ Does the child seem to be uncommonly nervous, as in projectile vomiting, bowel problems, etc.?

❥ Are there any bruises or marks or talk of the baby falling, being dropped, or of another child in the family hurting the new baby?

The presence of any or all of these signs may be the only warning flags that can alert a physician, other medical professional, or in some cases, a family member or friend to an ongoing case of PPD or PPPD prior to a fatal tragedy.

In my experience, there are often early signs of abuse such as the child being brought to a hospital or doctor with an elaborate story about "falling." Pediatricians in emergency rooms all over the country have reported their suspicion of abuse or neglect. X-rays taken in these instances clearly tell the tale of numerous fractures and broken bones, healed without medical treatment. But most of these cases are not followed up by the authorities after elaborate explanations by parents or family members have ameliorated those concerned individuals at the hospital. The system just isn't sufficient to make sure that each and every child and family is followed up on in the future.

After the hospital staff, next in line to help may be the marital counselors. These professionals are in a position to observe if the mother or partner is complaining that the other not helping enough, and/or that they have has no respite from the caretaking, or that family involvement is increasing the stress and strain.

THE MOTHER'S RELATIONSHIPS

Many relationships fall apart after the birth of a baby. The parents may be arguing or fighting. There may be complaints that the mother is not able to sleep and is constantly involved with worrying about baby, or totally unable to integrate her husband or significant other into the new home situation. Conversely, a therapist may hear from a family member that the mother is unable to care for the child, either because of fear of touching or harming the child, or because she is suffering from over-sleeping or is staying in bed most of the time.

Are there alcohol or drugs involved? If mother or partner has had an addiction problem before, has it reemerged?

Of course, if the family is not getting help from a counselor, then the neighbors, families, friends and finally, even the police may have to become involved. In cases where abuse becomes apparent or when the mother's problem finally comes to the attention of those around her, then it may be the authorities or even Health and Human Resource Service (HRS) who help in trying to resolve the conflict.

Often the couple and the family would like to find excuses for the erratic behavior. Common thoughts or statements indicating this type of denial include:

- "He/she must be jealous of the baby."
- "She doesn't have time for him/her anymore, she's so busy with the baby."
- "She's too tired to have sex or even be affectionate."
- "Poor thing, he/she has to work so hard and still stays up with the baby all night."

A healthy relationship certainly doesn't fall apart with the birth of a child. On the other side of the coin, even a healthy relationship can become strained if the mother's behavior is being influenced by an untreated mood disorder such as PPD. If the mother is suffering from a postpartum depression, she may be unduly preoccupied with her baby, or overly worried, abnormally angry, or detached. All of these symptoms should be looked at closely with postpartum depression in mind.

Despite previous notions that postpartum depression is prevalent only in certain segments of the population, it is now acknowledged that infanticide crosses racial, cultural, and socioeconomic lines. It's not black, Hispanic, Asian, Native-American, or white; it's not rich or poor. PPD, PPPD, and the infanticide cases that sometimes occur as a consequence of the illness when it is left untreated, does not discriminate.

If all else fails, families, friends, or perhaps the mother herself, should be sufficiently informed about the possibility of a postpartum depression if she is at risk or has the predisposition to be a candidate in light of her family history. Simply because forewarned is forearmed, families should be aware that any new behaviors should be scrutinized.

5 | PARTNERS

The narrator is a woman who has been taken to the country by her husband in an effort to cure her of some undefined illness—a kind of nervous fatigue. Although her husband, a doctor, is presented as kindly and well meaning, it is soon apparent that his treatment of his wife, guided as is by nineteenth-century attitudes toward women is an important source of her affliction and a perhaps inadvertent but nonetheless vicious abettor of it.—Elaine R. Hedges, from the Afterword of Charlotte Perkins Gilman's *The Yellow Wallpaper*[37]

RESEARCH SHOWS THAT a significant number of mothers who kill their children do so with the help of a partner. In fact, sometimes the partner or significant other is the actual killer. The tendency for people with mood disorders to gravitate toward a partner who has similar problems amplifies the condition of a mother with progressive postpartum depression. Therefore, it is important to speak of interdependency relationships in order to understand how both people play roles in the tragedies. Many of the cases I have studied involved not only a husband or boyfriend, but sometimes a female lover, a stepmother, or even a grandmother.

Even if they are not actually contributing directly to the problem, husbands, boyfriends, and significant others always play an important role in the postpartum picture. After all, pregnancy is also a significant precipitating life event for fathers and grandparents. Happy couples who wanted a child, celebrate the occasion. Even an unwanted pregnancy can evoke a feeling of pride in the mind of the father. With this in mind, the ensuing events surrounding a mother's postpartum depression become more complex and thus, are even more difficult to understand.

According to a 1982 article in *American Journal of Orthopsychiatry*, in one study, Drs. Davenport and Adland found a fifty percent incidence of mood instability episodes among 40 bipolar males during or immediately after their wives' pregnancies.[38]

Judging by recent newspaper reports, we find also that the partner may take on an alter ego role of the mother (i.e., acting for her, becoming the murderer or the abuser) with little or no interference from the depressed and vulnerable mother.

Marjory Fisher, bureau chief of the Queens (New York) district attorney's Special Victims Bureau, who has prosecuted child abuse cases for more than 12 years, says that in many of those cases, a mother's male companion had killed the child, but the mother either did not intervene or tried to cover up for the partner.

In several cases, women who have been beaten themselves or who have watched their children being beaten were too intimidated by their significant other to protect the children. In other words, most of the cases I investigated which included the involvement of a partner indicated a depression in the mother so profound that she was unable to intervene or protect the child from the partner. In these instances, not only is the mother incapacitated by the depression and her fears, but the partner as well as the child (or children) is deprived of her comfort and nurturing.

Without the mother's active participation in the family's care, the partner tends to become angry and frustrated, and then may act out his anger and displeasure over the interruption in their lives by taking it out on the child.

As stated previously, the tendency for individuals who have an affective disorder or the predisposition to mood disorders is to seek each other out. This is called "assortative mating."[39] The study describing this phenomenon states that two individuals, both prone to mood disorders, tend to be attracted to each other, increasing the probability of an eventual tragedy. The partner might be somewhat impaired, or at least prone to imbalance much of the time. Only a destabilized, unbalanced, confused woman could passively tolerate such dangerous and extreme behavior in a relationship. What help, after all, can two people in such condition be to each other in a time of stress?

My theory on the connection involved in partnerships in which is based on dependency issues. These couples, because of their own insecurities, tend to get into what I refer to as an 'inter-dependency' relationship as opposed to a more healthy 'mutual dependency' relationship.

I describe and illustrate this type of relationship using what I call my Domino Theory (see Figure I, A and B, below)

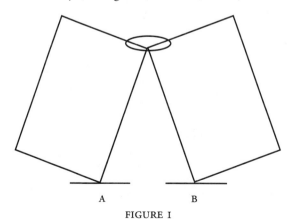

A   B

FIGURE I

Inter-dependency is the type of relationship I refer to when I speak of "partners in crime." The two dominos, which symbolize the two people, have gotten together because they have something in common. Each one is standing on one little point of his or her identity and stability (see A and B in Figure I, above). Neither one is well balanced and consequently they have what I call "glumped" on to each other out of necessity. And out of necessity, they must stay locked in that position. A is afraid to move because B might fall and B is in the same position—unable to straighten up, and the two remain out of balance and stuck.

It is also interesting to note that the extent of the crux relationship is at the point, where they actually touch (marked with an oval in the design). It is this one little point leaning on one spot which inevitability evolves, as it becomes painful, into a 'hostile dependency' relationship.

Imagine a defenseless child entering such a tense, precarious relationship. The family system would look something like this (see Figure II, below):

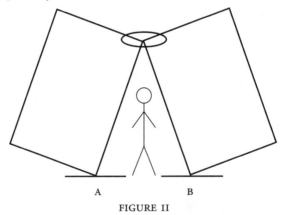

A   B

FIGURE II

It seems, then, in many of the cases in which the significant other commits the crime, that the mother, in her depression and hopeless dependency, unable to mobilize herself, fearful, unclear in her thinking, becomes a helpless bystander to the abuse and sometimes the murder of her child.

This dynamic was present in the case of the beating to death of seven-year-old Christina Holt by John Zile, her stepfather, enacted in front of her mother, Pauline Zile. The famous Zile case in Florida had two interesting components: 1) brutal abuse from John Zile, the child's stepfather and 2) an elaborate cover-up story, usually associated with *only* the mother's actions. The case occurred soon after the Susan Smith case, another case involving an elaborate cover-up. The Zile case came to trial during the writing of this book. Pauline was sentenced to life. John, the stepfather, has also been convicted.

The Zile case was in the headlines for a long time. To give you an idea of the notoriety this case received, 189 prospective jurors were interviewed. Out of that number, only five people said they had never heard about Zile or his dead stepdaughter.

While it was John who was charged with murder, prosecutors say although Pauline did not beat Christina on the night of her death, she abused her daughter in other ways, and she failed to protect her from John. John told police that he was punishing Christine for lying and soiling her pants.

Let's look at Pauline and her background. She had moved to Florida, leaving behind many problems—including a history of drug and alcohol abuse, a failed marriage, and Christina, then a baby girl, who went to live with relatives. She married John and had two more children over a five-year period. At the time of Christine's murder, Pauline was pregnant with a third child by Zile when Christina unexpectedly arrived on the doorstep of their crowded apartment, sent back to her by relatives. As tensions in the household increased, Christina was singled out for discipline that the other children did not have to endure.

Pauline was described by her attorney as emotionally weak and fearful of her husband, whom she said had beaten her. The attorney remarked, "Some people are strong and some people are not. What kind of mother is going to watch her daughter being beaten to death? No mother would do that. She was sound asleep when the beating started."

The attorney also stated that he would use a battered-woman defense. He said John controlled his wife, using the family's food money to buy marijuana.

"Also," the attorney said, "he convinced her to attempt suicide." Pauline and John had a suicide pact planned and they attempted to put it into action right before they were charged. It was a failed attempt, botched after trying to kill themselves with carbon monoxide poisoning. "He kept getting out to check the hose, getting fresh air, and she was in the car getting none," the attorney said. The car finally ran out of fuel and they were pulled over by police around 4:00 a.m. on their way to a service station for more. There was no suicide note.

To summarize the background surrounding the case: Pauline Zile was a woman displaced by moving from her family, who had a history of depression, was unable to care for her first child, and subsequently married John, an unstable, dysfunctional man, with whom she had two more children. Essentially, the stage of the Zile case was set with nearly every warning sign that might have alerted an outsider—a physician, family member, friend, or counselor—to the possibility of domestic violence.

Did Pauline at no time attempt to protect her child from the punishment which led to her death? Depression, by clinical description, is a feeling of hopelessness, a loss of energy, a loss of libido, a loss of appetite, a loss of interest in life. In Pauline's case—punctuated by her confusion, depression, and desperation—she saw the child as a detriment to having a life with the man she wanted. Like many women who either kill their children or do nothing to stop their partners from killing them, Pauline's background was fraught with symptoms and family traits strongly associated with depression. I picture her suicidal, despondent, sitting by watching her bully of a husband systematically "disciplining" her daughter, whom he considered the "problem" in their marriage, until little Christina Holt was dead.

The main point I'd like to highlight through this case is that to avert a tragedy, it is essential for at least one partner to be "healthy" or at least relatively stable. Without that, anything disastrous can happen and usually does, as in the case known as "Baby Lollipops."

In 1991, Lazaro Figueroa, age three, nicknamed by the newspapers as "Baby Lollipops" (because of the lollipops on the boy's teeshirt), was found under a bush in Miami Beach, Florida, beaten to death. Little Lazaro was malnourished and weighed only 18 pounds.

"It was the worst case of abuse and neglect I'd ever seen," says homicide detective Joe Matthews, now retired from the Miami Beach Police Department.[41] Among the boy's injuries was a fractured skull, which was determined to be the actual cause of death. Additionally, his right arm had been severely broken and healed without medical care. Burn marks scarred his body and toxicology reports showed insecticide and cocaine in his system. According to Detective Matthews, his disposable diaper had been taped to his body for about three months.

Police eventually arrested Anna Cardona, the mother, for the murder. She confessed after her 10-year-old son admitted his mother killed his little brother. His mother and her lover were convicted of the crime. Anna is serving a life sentence.

Both the Zile case and the "Baby Lollipops" case dramatically illustrate how essential it is for the mother with a mood disorder to be treated after the birth of her child. A mother whose postpartum depression is being treated and is free of depression can assure her partner that she is in charge and can balance her and her child's life with or without a partner. With treatment, the Domino Theory of a 'mutual dependency' would look like this (see Figure III, below):

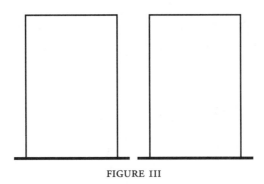

FIGURE III

As depicted in Figure III, a mutual dependency involves two people who stand on their solid bases, are autonomous, and are not unduly affected or suggestible to their partner's mood instability—at least not to the detriment of their child or children. They are stable and not fearful of sharing their feelings and fears with each other in order to have mutual understanding and support.

A treated person with a mood disorder produces an intact individual who can think clearly and act responsibly. She can regain her balance and stand solidly. A healthy mother feeling independent and autonomous could not stand by and watch her child or children abused or hurt in any way.

We know that women who grow up in violent homes not only learn to accept or tolerate violence, but also to expect it in their own interpersonal relationships. They have incorporated a kind of learned helplessness and passivity into their behavior. If they do, in fact, come from such a background, they typically learn the traditional sex roles in which boys are aggressive and girls are passive and submissive. Also they have learned that the male is considered patriarchal and maintains his will through dominance, coercion, and control.

The essential thing to remember is that disturbing trends and patterns like the ones outlined above do not abate during pregnancy or the postpartum period. In 1992, the U.S. Surgeon General, Dr. Joycelyn Elders noted that 62 percent of women in abusive relationships have suffered physical abuse during their pregnancies. This foreshadows future events for children involved in these relationships.

An unstable woman is also prone to abnormal jealousy, sometimes even of her own child. And in some instances, a father's obsessive attention to a child can also exacerbate this same irrational type of jealousy in his mate. In the November 14, 1994, issue of *Time,* Robert Hazelwood, a former FBI behavioral scientist, related an extreme manifestation of this abnormal behavior pattern when he described the case of a woman who became jealous of the attention her husband showered on their infant. One night, she told her husband she was cooking a roast for dinner. When he raised the cover, she said, "You love her so much, here she is."[41]

On the other side of the coin, in many cases, it is the mother's obsessive attention to her child that fosters animosity between partners. Regardless of which partner is more apt to be the source of violence against a child, in cases involving a deep depression in the mother, she is unable in many cases to protect the child from either her partner or from herself. The feeling of hopelessness, the loss of energy, the loss of libido, loss of appetite, loss of interest in life—all symptoms of a clinical depression—make the mother remain detached from whatever violence may transpire. She becomes a helpless onlooker of the partner's ire, almost like looking through a darkened mirror, detached and zombie-like.

Dr. Michael Durfee, a child psychiatrist with the Los Angeles County Department of Health Services, and a leading expert in the area, believes that men (usually the mother's partner) are more often responsible than women for killing offspring over the age of 12. This contention is borne out by state and local statistics. Durfee and other experts agree that the younger the victim, the greater the chance that his or her mother is the murderer. Certainly in the cases where there is a "partner in crime" involved, we can be aware of the mother being so seriously impaired as not to be able to prevent her child or children from being harmed by someone else.

During these times, the relationship between the mother and her partner grows extremely precarious, with the partner looking for logical explanations for the mother's behavior. The stability of the partner is of utmost importance because, without good judgment, the mother may be suspected of laziness and/or incompetence; family members may become critical, and view her as a "bad mother."

The partner's role becomes even more important if there is a severe depression which may result in hospitalization or even incapacitation. This could continue to be a problem during the time of recovery from treatment, whether it is done on an in- or outpatient basis.

The increased stresses certainly will involve increased responsibility in the home, especially when there are other children. There will be greater anxiety regarding the demands and needs of those children.

What about the unmet sexual needs of the partner? Will they not color the thinking and attitude of the partner? All of these issues, conflicts, and rapid changes will envelop the mother, child, and partner in a cloud of frustration. Certainly the issue of increased financial pressure will enter the picture as well.

The partner and/or family members will be suffering from frustration, anger, rejection, and resentment. It is at these times that we see inappropriate behavior manifested by the partner or significant others, which may well evolve to abuse of the newborn or other siblings.

The interview below of a mother we will call "Cheryl Stone" is one of the most moving and comprehensive cases I encountered which illustrates these factors all too well. Cheryl was a corporate wife, the mother of four children, who came from a family of professionals and was active in her church and community. She lived several hundred miles from her parents, sisters, and brothers, with whom she spoke and visited regularly. When Cheryl murdered her husband and youngest baby, the entire family and community were shocked.

The following is Cheryl's story in her own words:

"I had dated my husband for several years before we got married, and we were married for 10 years. So we had been together for a long time, and were happily married. We had a normal life—he was a business man and I was a homemaker. I was a physician's assistant before we had children.

"We began having a family after three years of marriage. Even though there were no circumstances outside of my life to cause me to have symptoms of depression, I was just depressed. I had every reason to enjoy life, but I wasn't. I had had a low level of depression throughout my life, but was never treated for it. I was still functional. I was just suffering from not wanting to live and not having enjoyment from life.

"Eventually this feeling became chronic. It was the kind of depression where I didn't want to get out of bed in the morning. Just fatigued all the time and just didn't have any enjoyment. For no reason. I mean, I had everything any person could ever want—in a marriage, in a husband. He was wonderful. He took care of me. He made a good living and we had a beautiful home and family. You know, you couldn't ask for anything more.

"My husband could never understand it—he was exactly the opposite from me—flamboyant and very active in the community. Nevertheless, he was very tolerant of my moods and my depression.

We figured it was just a mild depression—not something that required professional help. After all, I was functional. And I was still able to participate in my children's activities in school.

"My mother had had hormone problems, and they gave her hormones to balance out her chemistry. When I was a teenager, I went to all kinds of endocrinologists to find out about myself, and why I wasn't having periods. From the time I was about 12 years old. I was very irregular. I would have a period once a year. So I attributed a lot of my depression to the hormone imbalance. They gave me all kinds of options, like taking the pill [birth control pills]. But since I smoked, I didn't want to take the pill. I had a grandparent who had had cancer and who committed suicide, not wanting to put the family through the pain and suffering of her illness.

"The doctors even mentioned surgery, but I wasn't interested. When I got married, I was unable to get pregnant. It was three years into the marriage, during my routine evaluations, that we found out that I was pregnant.

"It was not a very normal pregnancy, and my baby was born prematurely. She was born with a disability and was in the hospital for five months when she was born. She only weighed less than one pound, but that's a whole other story. I don't know whether I suffered postpartum depression the first time or whether it was the serious problems the baby had.

"The worst time was after my third child. Although the pregnancy was normal, I had severe depression.

"It was after the fourth baby that I began to have some symptoms. After the first and second children, I only suffered a mild depression. They were three years apart. There were two years between my second and my third. And 16 months later, I got pregnant with my fourth.

"We had a wonderful marriage—we communicated. The main problem that I had was low self-esteem. I thought I was a bad mother. I think that the real postpartum symptoms were the swings I didn't recognize in myself. For no reason at all I would get very irritable and I was always tired.

"I had bad thoughts about myself as a mother and I wanted to protect my children from myself, and any harm that I could do to them psychologically, emotionally. I was saying things I couldn't believe I was saying. After the words came out of my mouth, I thought why am I saying these things? Sometimes they were very cruel things.

"My husband was out of town between the second and third pregnancies, when I had a miscarriage. That was a bad scene. I was saying things I could not believe I was saying to him. He was a very faithful husband. I was paranoid. It was a nightmare.

"After the third child, I started crying for no reason. I came to the point where I couldn't even function. My husband finally called somebody to get me in to see a doctor. It was a psychologist and she recommended that I see a psychiatrist in order to get on some medication. So that was the first time I was on medication.

"They gave me a commonly used anti-depressant, new on the market. After a month I was stabilized. It was like night and day. My attitude changed. I had never seen life as light and as wonderful as it was at that time. The medicine just changed my whole outlook on life. It was the first time I had really enjoyed life. So I stayed on it until I got pregnant again.

"I got off the medication because of the pregnancy. Everything was fine but I was really emotional through all my pregnancies. My moods were clearly up and down constantly throughout all my pregnancies. My husband always wanted to ship me off, I was so difficult. After my fourth one, remember, I hadn't been on the medication, and I went back to another psychologist.

"About a month or two after my fourth child was born, I went back on the anti-depressant medication. [But] I noticed the baby becoming irritable after breast-feeding, so I took myself off of the medication myself, without consulting a doctor. I guess that it was a bad decision, but I didn't want to harm him through the breast milk.

"There was nobody to inform me. I didn't have the education beforehand. I didn't know what to do. I was running around like a bandit. All I wanted to do was to get the kids out of my care. I mean, the faster they could get out of my care, the better, because I didn't want to harm them. Not physically. I just didn't want to hurt them emotionally. I really felt horrible as far as being a mother. I felt like the worst person. Why was God doing this and allowing me to have these children when I was such a horrible mother?

"I ended up not taking medication for five months. Then, I thought maybe if I started seeing a counselor, it would help. It was a pastoral counselor and he was more of a spiritual and religious counselor.

"I think he really didn't recognize what I was telling him and that what had happened might have had some medical basis. He wanted to put it into a spiritual context, which only fed more into my fears and delusions. I had started having a lot of delusions.

"The kids each had their places they could go, except for the baby—the youngest. I remember one time specifically, I had a late afternoon appointment with the counselor and they were home. I had gotten a baby sitter. My second little girl was five at the time. She said: 'Mommy, I want to go with you.' and 'Mommy, don't go.' I said, 'Mommy's got to go. She's going to learn to be a better mother.' And it was like she really understood after I told her what I was trying to do—that I was going to get help. I was seeking help as much as I could. I knew something was wrong, but I didn't know what to do about it. I was going literally—crazy—out of control.

"My husband had gone with me to the counselor the first time. He noticed a change in me after I started seeing the counselor. It actually seemed as if I was getting better. What was really happening was that I was going from the depressed stage into a hypo-mania where I started having more energy. So the irony is that while I seemed to be getting better, I was actually getting worse. And, of course, nobody recognized it.

"...the week prior to what happened, I had been in touch with my mother. I talked to her every day to keep close contact with her. During the time when I went into an actual manic state, which I had never really been in before, I didn't call her—any day. And she didn't call me because she felt she didn't want to bother me, that I was busy. So nobody was recognizing what was going on. My husband didn't realize what was going on. I wasn't sleeping properly. I wasn't sleeping at all. I didn't sleep for four days. I didn't eat anything for four days—I didn't feel as though I needed to.

"I was dancing and singing—not that I can carry a tune—but I was singing. I guess I thought I had the ability and power to do anything.

"It was all building up and I didn't know. We were getting ready to go on vacation the next day. My daughter who was born prematurely and with a disability, was ill.... I wanted desperately for her to be able to be healed. We were going to an island, a beach, and I wanted her to be able to enjoy the ocean, so I was going to pray for her to be healed. I went to pray for her, and she said, 'Mommy, you need the trumpet piece,' which was a piece from one of her toys and it was in the attic. I got my husband out of bed, and said, 'You have to go up in the attic and get that piece, because I praying for Paula, and she said I need that piece.' It was all very strange.

"He went up and got it and I prayed, and she didn't miraculously get well. I think that snapped me into a major mode of paranoia where I thought there was evil in the house. My husband was trying to calm me down, because I was frantic—I had lost it. One split second and it was over. He was trying to hold me down and stop me, calm me down. I saw a knife on the counter and I just grabbed the knife and then that was it. I stabbed him and my [baby] son."

"My son was on the floor in the kitchen. I had gotten him out of his crib and put him on the floor in the kitchen and he was crying. There was no thought that provoked me to do it that I can remember anyway.

"It was like a blackout. After it happened and the police got there—wait, I think my husband was calling the police. He got to the phone and called 911 and that's when I got the knife. I ended up cutting the phone cord, but they got the number before that, so they were on their way.

"...my baby was six months old when that mania happened. People don't associate postpartum symptoms with children of that age. They normally think of three to six weeks.

"I understand that the *New England Journal of Medicine* now acknowledges the condition as a total entity of its own, one that can last a year or more.

"That was what I went through as a part of what happened to me.... I was incarcerated and then I had to be seen by psychiatrists and tested up one side and down the other. I didn't have a clue that what was happening was mania.

"The whole state of mind after it happened was unreal. I couldn't believe it. It was like coming and going in and out of reality. I would realize what happened and I would go back into a delusional state. I was actually having hallucinations of seeing things that weren't really there.

"People don't understand or even see it—that's where all the 'I'm going crazy,' or 'You're driving me out of my mind'... types of phrases come from. They are very real and I didn't acknowledge the reality of them until after that happened. No one seemed to know that there was something wrong. Except the pediatrician, who was the only one who recognized what he called 'distraction' when I came in with the baby for a check-up.

"When the police came, they took me to jail. Fingerprinted me. Now I know that all the other children saw the whole thing. They weren't asleep. The whole house was in an uproar, because of the energy levels. I was wild.

"So they took me into the jail and evaluated me there and then took me into the hospital. I was there for six months. Then they sent me to the state hospital, where I stayed for almost two years and I underwent all kinds of tests. They did an MMPI and all kinds of tests, even a CAT scan in the emergency room. I don't think they tested for a chemical imbalance.

"I think a lot more women who suffer from those things and are coming forward. I met other women in the hospital who have had similar stories.

"As I look back, when I didn't feel happy about events, I always attributed it to my depression. By the time all this happened, I realize now, I had a full blown bipolar disorder.

"This happened six years ago. Since then, I have been in a State Hospital for all that time and then I went into a residential program. I was one of the more fortunate ones, to be able to get out of the system. I'm not out of the mental health system. I don't mean it that way, but I'm not in a half-way house, where they don't really take care of the people's actual problems and they don't get the help they really need.

"I am fortunate and blessed to be able to have afforded a lawyer and to get the support that I really needed. I have been able to see doctors and counselors and to be put on medicine. I'm on tons of medicine—an anti-convulsant medication for mood stabilization, an anti-depressant and an anti-psychotic I hope to get off of after I'm completely stabilized.

"...I now believe that chemicals are the basis for these reactions to hormonal changes, especially to stress. If you're under a lot of stress, it changes your biochemistry, just like with diabetes. If someone with the condition exercises more than normal or has added stress, they have to adjust their insulin. They start to have behavioral changes. A lot of the behavior is mistaken for socially unacceptable behavior. In my case, criminal. People don't understand it's impact and how it plays in the whole scheme of things."

Cheryl's account makes her predisposition to serious postpartum depression seem obvious. Yet no one around her seems to have recognized or acknowledged it—not her husband, her mother, sisters or brothers, not even her pediatrician, who only noticed she was "distracted." Even her counselor "didn't know enough to know."

Cheryl's mother recalls, "I knew the stress she was dealing with. I would come back from visiting her and say, 'She's going to have a nervous breakdown.' One of her children was at the terrible two stage and everything was 'No, no, no.' The baby needed attention and then there were all the special demands of her oldest daughter, [the child] with the disability.

"To my knowledge, Cheryl had never been depressed in her early life. Everyone has looked for predisposition and we haven't found any one. I do have a family member who is an alcoholic, but that doesn't apply. And her grandparent on her father's side—a man's man and a woman's gentleman—the first thing he did when his feet hit the floor was have a drink and he kept drinking all day.

"I didn't know she had been on an anti-depressant. Neither [Cheryl nor her husband] wanted me to know that. If she had shared some of that with me, it might have been a different story. We have family members who are doctors. If we had known some of this, perhaps we could have done something.

"After all, she had an obstetrician and a pediatrician and was out in public where some could have noticed how frantic she was becoming. I say it was from having too much to do. She was involved in volunteer work of various kinds in the community besides everything else she had to do at home.

"I stayed with them after the birth of each child. I worked harder in her house than in my own. She seemed all right when I was there. It wasn't until six weeks after the birth, after I'd left, that the depression started. She didn't have family around her to take the pressure off.

"Her husband was a great father and a good husband when he was there. [However] even at nine o'clock [in the evening] he often wasn't home. He was working his way up the corporate ladder and was on many local boards. He was a community leader. Often he was not home to help put the children to bed or anything else. On top of that, he traveled.

"She was so manic that she was dancing and singing that night [of the stabbing]. She and I usually talked every day and when she didn't call I knew something was wrong. I didn't hear from her for four days.

"The night this happened a relative was talking to her on the phone. He called her and found her babbling in a manic state. He said, 'If you don't stop this, I'll come out there.' He knew something was ghastly wrong that night. It was the first indication."

This tragedy as told by both Cheryl and her mother illustrates the vital importance of support, not only from the standpoint of being helpful, but also in acting as an intelligent observer of the mother's state of mind and behavior. These observers can then interpret the mother's condition to the rest of the family. They have the opportunity to notice that "something is wrong" and perhaps even intervene. It is during this crucial period that information is essential. Even if the family and friends don't correctly understand the mother's behavior—their observations will be critical. The case of "Cheryl Stone" depicts the mysterious beginnings of this tragic entity: The symptoms waxed and waned, sometimes seeming to be better for brief periods, but then followed by short-lived spells of erratic, sometimes even manic, behavior. What Cheryl evolved to was full blown manic-depression. Though she had had depressions in the past, she finally expressed a mania, which then clearly could be diagnosed.

Cases like that of Cheryl Stone reveal that even though a mother may seem to rally and begin to assume some of her responsibilities, she may still be suffering from the underlying depression, which has only abated for the time being. Unsuspectingly, any trigger may launch her into a renewed state of depression. These symptoms could well mark the beginning of the cycle of progressive postpartum depression. The long 'mild' depression Cheryl describes, untreated for so long, was exacerbated by the birth of each successive child, resulted in full blown manic-depressive illness (bipolar disorder) and the subsequent psychosis leading to the tragedies.

Whether mother's depression is mild or severe, it affects her entire environment. Family and friends are involved as well as siblings, by virtue of her diminished capacity to care for herself, her child, and her partner. In our society there is an expectation that the word "mother" connotes a "caretaker." If she is unable to fulfill those duties, everyone around her is affected: The abandonment felt by a partner and the other children, the disappointment by grandparents in her lack of joy, and the mother's own energy level (agitated, diminished, or increased) all invoke anxiety and fear. Certainly this is a time when all relationships may suffer from increased stress and strain.

In some cases involving family members who have assumed the role of caretaker to the new baby while the mother is being treated for postpartum depression, the family members may lose confidence in the mother's ability to care for her child. Subsequently, they may be reluctant to return the baby to the mother or allow her to assume her natural responsibility. This hesitation can frighten and demoralize the mother, who then grows reluctant to share her pain and fears. Both the mother and the family become concerned about the stigma. They may feel that it will follow them, long after treatment is over. Unfortunately, the shame and embarrassment of not being viewed as a "good mother" prevents treatment in many cases.

Overprotectiveness by family members is a double-edged sword. When the mother is ill and unable to function at full capacity, she and the baby need extra attention. But many times the family's trust has been affected and they are reluctant to give up their various roles in the care of the child or children. Here especially more education, support, and understanding are vital.

6 | MOTHERS WHO KILLED

Our first impulse is that something almost unimaginably evil has occurred. But far from unimaginable, the murder of very young children by their mothers is, and always has been, among the most common forms of homicide; and whether these cases involve evil or mental illness or represent an indictment of the social conditions of women's lives is a legal and philosophical problem of great complexity.—Daniel Maier-Katkin, Dean of the School of Criminology and Criminal Justice at Florida State University[42]

USUALLY ONLY THE most sensational cases capture the attention of the public. Of these "headline cases," we find the same common factors that go unpublicized from private medical practices. Given the numerous cases of child abuse, murder, and tragedies in the news, why are we not insisting on scientific investigations about the cause? The information is available, yet still not widely disseminated. Each time another headline story appears regarding a mother killing her children, the public reacts with the same repeated incredulity.

What do cases of mothers who kill their children have in common? Not geography. Not age. Not ethnicity or race. Not class background. Not diet. One characteristic continues to emerge in cases in which it is the mother who perpetrates the crime against her own child—an elaborate cover-up concocted by mother and sometimes in collusion with her partner. For example, Susan Smith (the South Carolina woman referenced in previous chapters), prior to the discovery that she had killed her two sons, desperately pleaded on television to find the "culprit" who absconded with her children in her own car. Pauline Zile similarly beseeched the public to help her find her little daughter who "disappeared in a flea market."

THE BIG COVER-UP

In a November 5, 1994 editorial by Susan Weiner, a special contributor to the *Miami Herald,* Richard J. Gelles, a professor of sociology and psychology at the University of Rhode Island and an expert on family violence is quoted as saying, "about 700 mothers kill their children each year, and about 50 fabricate tales of abduction." While it is true that hindsight always brings 20/20 vision, if this type of cover-up is so common, why is it then that the media and in turn, the general public, are so slow to question the elaborate cover-up tales even when they sound far-fetched and unlikely?

Dr. Charles Ewing, JD, Ph.D., an upstate New York psychologist who is writing a book on inter-family murders, offers the following answer: "We're willing to believe the stories because we don't want to believe the alternative. We don't want to believe that Susan Smith killed her own children." This attitude is worth highlighting because it depicts how deeply our societal denial runs with regard to even the possibility of postpartum depression, progressive postpartum depression, and the sometimes extreme consequences of these conditions being anything more than a freak occurrence.

The Susan Smith case fits perfectly into the patterns exhibited in many of these cases, especially with regard to the cover-up angle. It all started with Smith's emotional claim that her two children had been abducted. The contradictory headlines that ensued when it was discovered that Smith not only lied, but in fact, that she herself killed the boys, were numerous and speak strongly toward the controversy surrounding PPD and PPPD:

> "Expert says Susan Smith dreams of joining her sons."
> "Susan Smith was judged legally competent to stand trial on murder charges for drowning her two sons, but she will take her life at the first opportunity," a state expert reported.
> "Suicidal but sane," read another newspaper headline.

Psychological evaluations of Smith after she had been apprehended for the murders offered similar contradictions in the sense that it was clear that she suffered from serious mental problems and yet was still deemed mentally fit to be put on trial for the murders. Dr. Donald Morgan of the South Carolina Mental Health Department stated that "Smith suffers from severe depression and an adjustment disorder that causes her to have an emotional reaction to stress." He added, "If she got out of prison, she said she would take her life as rapidly as possible."

Morgan also said that although Smith could stand trial on the two murder charges against her, he recommended that she not be allowed to testify because she would ask for the death penalty if put on the stand. "She feels she deserves punishment and her desire would be not to continue living in prison," Morgan said.

Dr. Morgan conducted several examinations on Smith, including one just before the hearing. Following his examinations, Morgan concluded, "It's easy to make a mistake thinking that she's better than she is. She fantasizes about being reunited with her children. She also has crying spells and nausea and takes anti-depressants to combat intense feelings of hopelessness, sleepless, and worthlessness. She repeatedly stated that she didn't want her children to be 'without a mother.'"

This was the description of a woman who committed a crime that broke the hearts of the 10,000-member community of Union, South Carolina. One could ask why no one in her family, nor her friends, her husband, or her lover noticed her condition.

As with numerous other cases discussed and examined in this book, the key to trying to address why and how such a violent and tragic series of events could take place is to go beyond the newspaper headlines and the TV segments by digging deeper into Susan Smith's past to see whether any signs of Smith's condition were apparent in her background. As it turns out, Smith's actions were linked to long-term history of mental problems, an unsurprising discovery in light of what we know about the link between postpartum depression and women with a previous history of mental illness. Keeping in mind the traits we have discussed regarding 'who is at risk?,' we remember that Susan's biological father committed suicide. Susan's older brother, Scotty Vaughan, read a letter he wrote to Susan in prison after she asked him about their father, Harry Vaughan, and his suicide. The letter recalled their parents' stormy marriage, their father's violent behavior, and finally the night he shot himself. "I'll never forget the hurt, the pain I felt when she [their mother] told me Daddy was dead. Then I thought about you [Susan] and how hurt you would be," Vaughan read.

Susan also reportedly had been sexually abused, which certainly may have been a factor in her depressions, and in turn, in her violent behavior years later as an adult. Some children cope with a trauma like molestation by depersonalizing or dissociating from it, a strategy that many experts believe they carry into adulthood. According to Julie Blackman, Ph.D., a psychologist and forensic consultant in New York, these individuals may lack any form of empathy for their children, and are unable to see them as separate beings.

Additionally, like her father, Smith herself had a preoccupation with suicidal feelings from the time she was 13. As a young girl, she attempted suicide twice with overdoses of aspirins—once at age 13 and again, at 18.

Her brother, Scotty Vaughan, also went on to say his sister never lost her temper with her two sons, Michael, 3, or 14-month-old Alex. He said his mother, Linda Russell, had helped to care for the two boys during Smith's troubled marriage. As this paradoxical portrait of Smith as a loving, nurturing mother indicates, this case also fits the characteristics of mothers who kill their children to 'protect them.' Smith herself later said she "would rather know that my children were living in heaven than that someone was hurting or torturing them."

And finally, what was the trigger that made Smith snap? In 1917, Freud wrote of the tendency to have "too strong fixations to their love-object and to a quick withdrawal of object cathexis. Object choice is on a narcissistic basis."[43] This description sounds very much like Susan Smith's own explanation of why she killed her children. All of the events leading up to Smith's condition finally came to a head when, along with financial problems that had plagued her for years, her boyfriend broke up their relationship with the excuse that he didn't want to become a stepfather. This conclusive rejection was apparently "the final straw" for Susan Smith. She loved a man who said he would withdraw his love and/or commitment because she had children. Her clouded thinking, personal needs, and the anticipation of losing his love is a perfect example of Freud's observations of people suffering from a fixation.

Similar findings by Dr. Karl Abraham, one of the earliest physicians to write about formulating traits, offer further insight into the Susan Smith case. He described "the patients' abnormal character development and inability to maintain good relationships." These features, he speculated, were coupled with an ongoing sense of impending loss of objects, which produce a 'rageful' stance toward these objects and their inability to "gratify narcissistic demands."[44] While obviously this description was not written in reference to the Susan Smith case, it is easy to see how it applies; certainly it offers a further explanation for how Smith reacted to her conflicted situation.

Susan's condition would not have been a surprise to an alert clinician, especially one familiar with her and her family. Arlene Andrews, a professor of social work at the University of South Carolina, offered insight into why Smith herself did not seek help for her chronic emotional problems. Andrews testified that Smith was traumatized as a teenager by fears that she had damaged her family by telling school officials that her stepfather was molesting her. "She's a very lovable person, but she didn't think she was lovable. She also believes it's real important to look like you have no problems. She thinks that if you ask for help, you'll get in trouble," Andrews said.

DR. RANDELL ALEXANDER, a child abuse expert at the University of Iowa Medical School, believes that the more elaborate the story concerning the circumstances of the child's death, the more likely it is that the crime involves the mother.

For example, in Texas, Darlie Routier, age 25, was accused of killing her five- and six-year-old children in her family's upscale suburban home. Much like Susan Smith, she had an intricate cover-up story: Her story was that an outside perpetrator entered the house, injured her, and committed the murders while her husband was asleep with the youngest child, eight-month-old Drake.

Routier, who reportedly had been sleeping on a couch a few feet from the boys, claimed she awoke and saw a man dressed in dark clothing who fled toward the garage.

Prosecutors later said Routier killed five-year-old Damon and six-year-old Devon on June 6, 1996, because she was angry over family money problems and the weight she had gained during a recent pregnancy. They said she slashed herself in an attempt to fool police.

A jury took four hours to decide the fate of Darlie. They could have given her life imprisonment, but she received the death penalty instead. She was reported to be "stone-faced" upon hearing the verdict. The prosecutor's interpretation of this cold response was, "She's not going to give the satisfaction of showing a reaction."

In a February 26, 1997 interview on *PrimeTime Live*, Darlie's mother, mother-in-law, and husband all stated they felt she was innocent. However, Darlie's behavior following the crime, like that of so many other women like her, was paradoxical. She did not exhibit behavior typical of a grieving mother who has played no part in the deaths of her children. Greg Davis, assistant district attorney for Dallas, said that on Devon's seventh birthday, for example, there at the graveside, was a postmortem "birthday party with Darlie singing 'Happy Birthday' and spraying silly string."

"I was in disbelief," stated Davis.

A reporter later described Darlie as "miserable—in the depths of postpartum depression after her third son's birth." It is interesting to note how many of these crimes are committed after the third or fourth pregnancy, which supports the argument that the underlying mental condition is progressive, worsening over time if it goes untreated. In the Routier case, the reporter went on to point out that Darlie was also "distraught because her husband's $250,000-a-year computer business had fallen on hard times.... The prosecutor described her as a woman who was depressed, gained weight, suffering from postpartum depression, behind in the mortgage, and financially strapped."

Interestingly, in retrospect, the prosecutor's portrayal of Darlie as described above only supports the interpretation of her as a woman who was plagued by a progressive mental illness rather than as a cold-blooded criminal. More than a month before the murders Darlie had considered an overdose of pills. Her behavior had been erratic—she had suddenly decided to hold a tenth anniversary party at a hotel with 150 guests. In the month before the murders, she lost 10 pounds. The night of the murders she and her husband argued over expenses of the Jaguar and their boat. She had not been sleeping well, so she decided to sleep downstairs with the two older boys.

Darlie's diary entries similarly suggested that she was suicidal and expressed a desire to be forgiven for something she was about to do. She was later placed on a suicide watch in jail following her conviction for the murders.

The guilty verdict came even after she was staunchly defended by her husband, her mother, and several friends at her trial, who along with Darlie adamantly protested that she was innocent. At the trial, she took the stand and told the jurors, "I loved those children more than my life. I did not kill my babies."

Nevertheless, despite a host of signs suggesting that such a tragedy might occur, the recent birth of Darlie's new baby, sleeping upstairs with Dad when the murders took place, was not taken into consideration in the case, nor was Darlie's behavior after the birth of that child. Ironically, the background to the cases indicates that, as in the case of Susan Smith, Darlie's case fits not only the pattern of an elaborate cover-up, but also that of a progressive postpartum depression. Nevertheless, postpartum depression was not regarded as a significant issue in the trial even though the third child was only eight months old.

A CASE IN MIAMI, Florida also involved a similar "cover-up" story: Mabel Dominquez was a caring wife and a patient, mild-tempered mother of two. But police said the 23-year-old woman had finally succeeded in doing what she had tried several times previously: suffocating her month-old daughter. After the baby died, Mabel walked across a busy avenue and threw the infant into a nearby canal.

Mabel initially told police a story similar to that of convicted killers Susan Smith and Darlie Routier. She said two black men in a van tried to grab one of her two daughters—Lazara or Barbara—while they walked along a local street with her baby Natalie.

But after police pressed her throughout the day, her story changed twice. In one version, she said the baby fell out of the stroller as she pushed it down the stairs of her apartment building. Then she said she accidentally dropped that baby when the two-year-old began to cry in a bedroom. After noticing that the baby was not breathing, she said, she decided to walk to her in-laws' house 13 blocks away for help.

It took her five hours to finally tell the police the version they accepted. She confessed that she had pinched Natalie's nose and covered her mouth until the baby died. She said she then scratched her own chest and Lazara's legs to make her story look plausible. She admitted she had been feeling overwhelmed since the birth and had tried to kill the infant before.

"According to her, she had been depressed lately," said Sergeant Carlos Hernandez-Adan. "We don't know why." Again, although newspapers reports clearly stated 'the woman was depressed,' no one, it seems, made the connection between the mood, the event, and the subsequent action.

Shocked family and friends remembered a far different Mabel.

"I don't understand," said a longtime family friend. "She was a happy, active person. I was with her when she had the baby and was breast-feeding her. She was very happy."

A 1983 CASE IN OREGON illustrates another elaborate cover-up. Elizabeth Diane Downs claimed that a bushy-haired stranger waved down her car on a deserted road and shot her and her three children, killing seven-year-old daughter Cheryl Lynn. She reported it as an attempted kidnapping. Her seven-year-old daughter died, and her eight-year-old daughter and three-year-old son remain badly disabled.

Diane, as she was known, had been a surrogate mother and given birth almost one year to the day prior to the murders. She had given up the baby immediately to the new mother. Additionally, she had had an abortion between the births of her second and third children, a decision which she later regretted. In reference to her subsequent choice to be a surrogate mother for $10,000, Diane later gave the following statement in an interview: "People have wondered why I won't regret this, giving up the baby.... And that's very easy to answer. When you kill a child, when you have an abortion, you've terminated something. You've murdered somebody—it's cruel, it's horrible, it's terrible. But when you do something out of love, when you carry a child for somebody else, and turn that life over to them, you haven't done anything bad, and it's nothing you look back on and regret. It's good."

At the time of the murder, Diane was divorced from the father of her children and was dating a married man who she described in her diary as "not wanting to be a father," and for whom the children would be a burden. However, choosing between her boyfriend and her children was not the only conflict that led up to the murder. Like many of the other filicide cases, Diane's own early childhood history involved alleged sexual abuse at the age of twelve by her father and a history of mental instability, with an attempted suicide at age thirteen. Diane grew up in Arizona, the daughter of a postal worker. As a child, she didn't like her father's lectures, strict rules, and the power he had over her mother. Diane testified that when she was 12, he sexually abused her. When she was 13, she tried to cut her wrists. At 18, with a high school education, she married Steve Downs, a farmhand she described as being as dominating as her father.

Diane eventually gave birth to her first child, Christie, whom she called her "first good friend." Another daughter, Cheryl, was born the following year and was described as a colicky baby. She ended her next pregnancy with an abortion, but regretted doing so later after seeing pictures of fetuses at an anti-abortion booth at a local fair: "When I had the abortion, I was led to believe that a six-week fetus is nothing more than mucus."

After the birth of her third child, Danny, she still felt the loss. "I found you cannot replace a child that you have killed," said Diane during an interview with Elizabeth Bumiller of the Washington Post News Service.

The Diane Downs case has a familiar ring to it; the background events leading up to tragedy is remarkably similar to the events that preceded the Susan Smith case. First, both cases involved a possible history of early abuse by a father or father figure. Secondly, both women had made previous suicide attempts. Third, both women made emphatic statements that contradicting their violent behavior about how important the children were to them in their respective lives. Both women also used an elaborate cover-up story in order to hide their crimes. And, finally, both women were involved in new relationships in which the new boyfriend made it clear that he did not want her children in their lives. Entries in Diane's diary, contained statements (presumably addressed to her married lover) that reveal her conflicted emotions: "I still think of you as my best friend and lover, and you keep telling me to go away and find someone else," and "I'm a little sad that Charlene [a friend] has convinced you that the kids would be a burden, because I know it would not be true."

To add to the bizarre nature of the case, Henry Stern reported in a March 1989 Associate Press article entitled "Child-Killer Mother Plans to Rewed: Elizabeth Downs Maps Out Book, Marriage From Prison Cell" that Diane spent her time writing letters to her new fiancé, who saw her on *The Oprah Winfrey Show* and wrote to her because he felt sorry for her. In the interview, Diane described herself as "the most hated woman in America" and was also quoted as saying, "What happened the night of the shooting was so horrendous, so unexpected, so unbelievable. I'm very self-disciplined and I need to have control of my own existence. I just reached a point of not knowing what was real and what wasn't."[45]

As in the Susan Smith case, the Downs case emphasizes both the mother's self-denial as well as the denial of those around her as to the possibility of postpartum depression or especially progressive postpartum depression as a cause of the tragic outcome.

Diane Downs was convicted of murder and is serving a life sentence. The surviving children were adopted and a baby with whom she was pregnant at the time of the trial was given over to the state.

A GRANDMOTHER WHO KILLED

The very essence of this book is to reexamine our societal viewpoint regarding crimes like the ones described in this chapter. The use of an elaborate cover-up story is one common factor in many cases of mothers who kill their children. However, it may not be the most useful correlation in terms of promoting prevention and intervention. Perhaps the best *preventive* measure is an awareness of a mother's family history and mental health history by those who are in a position to recognize early signs of trouble and intervene before a murder occurs. All of the women described in this chapter—who were at risk, and clearly identified as such *after* violence had occurred—had the same capacity to love and care for their children as other women. If only they, their family members, friends, or doctors could have been forewarned to recognize the danger signs and family history, they could then have been treated before a disaster occurred and felt safe having children.

More attention needs to be paid to background history; as we can see by the tragic results in case after case in which early signs went unrecognized, early diagnosis of mental instability and possible illness is essential. When families, friends, the general public, and medical professionals become more cognizant of the mother at risk, prevention, caution, and intervention would occur *before* the crime.

Although it concerns a grandmother rather than a mother, the 1996 case in Florida of Christine Sharrow, 41, who killed her 19-month-old granddaughter, Alexandria, while babysitting, illustrates the necessity of a shift away from the way we currently regard these cases only as either inexplicable or aberrational acts of violence rather than part of a progressive condition.

Christine Sharrow described to *Miami Herald* journalist David Kidwell[46] that she wanted a relationship with her grandchild, a toddler. She said she and the baby had a loving, warm relationship. In her description of the crime, without emotion, she remembered their last hug, how she fed her Fruit Loops before scooping her up and strangling her with a bathrobe sash. "I don't remember feeling anything," the grandmother said. "My heart was stone." Sharrow also related that she had spent the several months prior to the murder in a fog induced by vodka.

After the murder, she lay the dead baby on her back in the kitchen freezer over the few remaining frozen dinners inside. In the interview with Kidwell, Sharrow said she strangled Alexandria "to save her from a life of neglect and depression." She now wants to fire her lawyers, plead guilty, and go to the electric chair: "...I don't want any help. I'm not making any excuses. I don't want my lawyers. I don't want their psychologists. I'm competent. I am now and I was then. I'm not insane. I just want to go to Death Row and save everybody a lot of time and money. I don't want to go on living with what I did."

When thoroughly examined, this particular case well describes the untreated progression of PPD in a woman who had been mentally ill throughout her life. It probably began after the birth of Sharrow's own son, with her first episode of bipolar illness. Her long-term history points to the fact that genetically she expressed the illness even before the birth of her own child, but was not treated.

Christine Sharrows' life was chaotic and troubled beginning as far back as her teens. During her first marriage at the age of 16, Sharrow was a victim of physical abuse and also suffered a miscarriage of twins. Divorce was not long in coming, but Sharrows was not single for long. She remarried at 18 and had three children. The marriage lasted eight years and ended in another divorce. Sharrows married a third time and was widowed after five years.

In the interview with Kidwell following the murder, Sharrow also talked about her own troubled life of alcoholism, manic-depression, and domestic violence. According to records, Sharrow had attempted suicide at least 18 times, been in and out of drug and alcohol rehabilitation, and spent almost three years in prison on a manslaughter conviction.

Despite this volatile past, little has been written about the fact that prior to the strangulation of Alexandria, Christine Sharrow had already been the subject of a complaint which had triggered an investigation by the State Department of Health and Rehabilitation. The caller told investigators that a child living at Alexandria's address had a bruised eye as well as bruises on her back. The call was eventually filed as a false complaint, but the murder followed shortly thereafter. At the time of her arrest, Christine accused Alexandria's parents of drug abuse and child neglect. Reports indicated that Sharrow felt her granddaughter would be better off dead.

Despite the fact that the perpetrator of the crime was a grandmother, the case has all the earmarks of the "mother killings" we are investigating. As Dr. Steven Shea of the University of South Carolina School of Medicine, outlined at the American Psychological Association's convention in 1995:

"...[in nearly all the filicide cases in which the murders are committed by the mother] methods of killing included beating the children with a blunt object, suffocating, arson, and drowning.... Early detection and treatment of mental illness in mothers is vital to prevent child abuse and infanticide... these women reportedly were undergoing stressful periods in their lives at the time. Yet most of them were not seeking treatment at the time of the crime."[47]

THE "UNPREDICTABLE" EVENT

Jill Korbin, an anthropology professor at Case Western Reserve University and author of a study of women incarcerated for deadly child abuse states, "These women often let others know about incidents of abuse prior to the fatal event. But many times, the seriousness of the incidents isn't recognized."

With headline cases like the ones cited in this chapter, we often know very little about the mothers' backgrounds and therefore, incidents of abuse are not regarded as part of an ongoing pattern. In this way, the women in these cases exemplify just how such mothers go undetected as prime candidates for postpartum depression or suicide. Other than the genetic predisposition, they often show no clues to the erratic behavior that precedes the crimes. I have included some cases here, despite their sketchy personal histories, in order to illustrate an atypical symptom. Mania is a symptom which may seem foreign to a postpartum depression, however, many mothers in these cases have manifested behaviors that were wild, hyperactive, agitated, unreasonably raging and angry, sometimes including inappropratie laughter—these are all symptoms of mania.

But whether or not these women did or did not have recorded psychiatric histories, in most cases, no one expected murder to be one of the symptoms. In most of these cases, their parenting skills, according to family members, seemed to reflect a caring and nurturing attitude, right up until PPD consumed and enveloped them in a cloud of unreality. It was at those times that the crimes occurred, which accounts for why they are seen as 'unpredictable' events. Given the myriad of vague and varied symtpoms, combined with erratic, shifting moods, it follows that strange behavior that occurs in conjunction with the 'blessed event' is usually overlooked as being temporary and concomitant with the new situation.

As Suzanne Barnard, a social worker with the children's division of the American Humane Association, says: "I don't think most parents who murder children wake up in the morning and say, 'This is the day I'm going to kill my kids.'" Certainly this statement speaks to the unpredictability of the homicidal action.

Dewey Cornell, a clinical psychologist at the University of Virginia states: "Usually one thing leads to another, and the problem escalates to the point where eventually the person caves in under the pressure and stress."

Dr. Cornell goes on to say, "Most typically this is in the context of a woman who is severely depressed and may also be suicidal." Other doctors are inclined to cite psychosis or sometimes, postpartum depression.

In my experience, I have come to similar conclusions, in that these women's actions were totally unpredictable, and sometimes paradoxical, in terms of their mothering skills, even if their biological or emotional histories point to postpartum possibilities. This has especially been true, as most of the cases I personally examined were women whose previous history or mothering skills were never in question.

A case in point is that of Donna Fleming, age 24. Having just found that she was pregnant again, she pushed a stroller with her two sons to the middle of the 50-foot-high Ocean Boulevard Bridge over the Los Angeles River and dropped them, one by one, over the side. Then she jumped. Donna and her three-year-old son survived. Twenty-month-old Craig Allen did not.

When a police officer arrived on the scene, Donna was screaming, "My kids! My kids!"

The officer stated that Donna acknowledged throwing the children off the bridge, then jumping in. She did not say if she was trying to kill herself. She was charged with murder and attempted murder.

When this incident took place, no one knew just how troubled Donna was at the time. Her husband of four years said he had no idea why his wife had done such a thing. However, neighbors and police told of a troubled marriage. Her husband was abusive and had been arrested and convicted several times over the preceding thirteen months for wife beating. Detectives revealed that Donna suffered minor injuries in some of the six reported attacks by her husband. Each time she refused medical care. The day of Donna's crime against their children was her husband's 37th birthday.

Apparently, however, prior to the murder, there was no questioning of Donna's parenting skills, in spite of the lifestyle she was leading and her multiple pregnancies, until the shocking actions took place. This is characteristic in most of the cases where the mother's genetic history has not been examined.

In a dissimilar and somewhat more predictable case of violent behavior, Ramona Perez fatally stabbed her nine-year-old son Rafael in the heart. Diagnosed with a psychiatric illness, her family feels that she had no idea what she was doing at the time she killed her son in front of his younger brother. Her sister and brother state that when Ramona was 20, she radically changed from a "loving big sister to a tormented stranger."

Ramona gave no explanation except that Rafael had been "mean" to her and to his younger brother. However, in the days preceding the stabbing, one of Rafael's friends said that Rafael told him "my mother's going to kill me." Perhaps her psychiatric history began when Rafael was born. In fact, in spite of Ramona's psychiatric history, she was thought to be a good mother by the boy's father who "never suspected his kids were in danger."[48]

MOTHERS WHO KILLED NEWBORNS

Numerous cases involving the murdering of newborns by the mothers, sometimes with the help of a partner, have appeared in the newspapers in recent years. The high frequency of teenage mothers as well as older mothers who have been found guilty of killing newborns is particularly disturbing. According to a CNN review of FBI statistics, for example, nearly five infants under the age of one are killed in the United States each week. The report contains the most recent information available and was based on 1995 data that showed 249 infants were killed that year.[49] The age of the mother aside, however, because most of the cases involving a killing almost immediately following birth tend to be reported only in local papers, there is less of a general and widespread impact on, in and turn response by, the general public. Isolating the incidents in the press in this way as purely 'local news' creates a skewed picture of the events and makes it harder to recognize these occurrences as part of a larger problem. However, even just a short national sampling like the list of cases I have researched and compiled below, taken from various local papers in different states across the U.S., relates the huge scope of the problem:

- Casselberry, Florida—People found a dead newborn wrapped in plastic bags in a closet and charged Mary Butler, 23, with killing the child a few hours after birth.

- Zion, Illinois—Lynn Zaworski, 19, allegedly suffocated her infant within an hour of the birth.

- Chicago, Illinois—Catika Grant, 16, was convicted of involuntary manslaughter and concealment of a homicidal death for allowing her newborn daughter to drown in the toilet minutes after she gave birth.

- Elgin, Illinois—The body of a newborn baby girl was found by police in the basement of the home of Catalina Andrade, 27. Andrade was charged with first-degree murder.

- Palatine, Illinois—Elizabeth Ehlert, 33, was charged with killing her newborn baby by placing the infant in a creek behind her home just minutes after the birth.

- St. Paul, Minnesota—Mary C. Leggate, 39, a mother of four, was convicted of first-degree intentional homicide. Leggate had been found guilty of placing her newborn daughter in a cardboard box and throwing it in a trash bin. Leggate was found to be legally sane and faces a mandatory life term.

- St. Paul, Minnesota—Michelle Buranen, 17, was accused of murdering her newborn child by repeatedly stabbing it and then burying it in a shallow grave in the back yard of her father's home. A psychologist involved in the investigation said Michelle had been exposed to alcohol abuse, physical aggression, and a chaotic life. Michelle was charged with first-degree murder and two counts of second-degree murder.

❧ Wichita, Kansas—Jean Franks, 19, strangled her newborn baby girl and threw the body into a trash can. She had pleaded not guilty by reason of insanity, claiming she suffered from psychological problems that prevented her from knowing the difference between right and wrong. She was put on probation for five years after being diagnosed by a psychiatrist with a dissociative reaction (a protective device that kept Jean from feeling any pain when the baby was born and blocked out her memory of the birth and the strangulation).

❧ Escanaba, Michigan—Connie Pendleton, 28, entered a plea bargain after being charged with murder for smothering her newborn son just after giving birth in a service station restroom. Pendleton claimed she had hidden her pregnancy and killed the baby because her boyfriend did not want children.

IN THE CASES OF teenage girls who hid their pregnancies, gave birth, and in a postpartum panic, did the unthinkable, and threw their babies away—in trash cans, dumpsters, or toilets—we must consider how clouded their judgment must have been. Was it related to the dramatic trauma of the birth itself of the unwanted child or to the strain of the denial given the secret these girls had successfully hidden for nine months? Did the hysteria or shock have that instant result? And how distorted was their cognition?

Interestingly, some experts who have commented on teenagers who gave birth secretly and immediately attempted to do away with the child chalked most of the problem up to immaturity and dependency on their parents. For example, according to Phillip Resnick, a professor of psychiatry at Case Western Reserve University who has studied the phenomenon: "[These women] may have denied their pregnancy, missed the opportunity for abortion and then passively feel that the situation will somehow take care of itself—that the infant will be stillborn."[50] Stephanie Coontz, a historian who has written about the changing role of families has made similar comments, saying "girls have been giving birth to babies and, terrified of what their parents or others might say or do, they've abandoned those babies to die or buried them alive or disposed of them in any way they could think of."[51]

Certainly a case could be made concerning the societal and sociological pressures surrounding a pregnant, unmarried teenager and her decision about the outcome of her pregnancy—her baby. However, since the act of murder erases an innocent life, it indicates a possible projection of the mother's own self-hate because of her inability to provide a decent life for the baby onto the baby itself. The element of depression and the lack of clear thinking are clinically termed "cognitive deficits."

As a professional, I find it difficult to accept that these murders are acts of pure selfishness and immorality, despite the fact that a teenager's immaturity may be a contributing factor. For why would one teenager give birth and put the baby in safe surroundings while another with no previous criminal history makes this heinous choice?

Like the other filicide cases I have cited, these cases are similar in nature—though none of the women knew each other or came from the exact same background—all seemed to act in the same irrational way.

On June 6, 1997, in Freehold, New Jersey, a high school senior, age 18, gave birth at her high school prom, then dumped the baby in the trash. Melissa Drexler was charged with murder and endangering the welfare of her child. According to Monmouth County prosecutor John Kaye, Melissa claimed her baby was born dead, but the autopsy revealed that the baby had been born alive and died from manual strangulation and asphyxiation. However, friend of Melissa defended her saying, "Melissa is not a bad person even though she did a bad thing. She's not one of those kids that has no regard for life." Even Prosecutor Kaye admitted that her behavior didn't mesh with the evidence that followed the investigation: "[Melissa] undoubtedly was frightened and upset. It just doesn't fit." In answer to those comments, psychologist Dr. Joyce Brothers said, "These are not bad kids, but kids who are so responsible and dependent emotionally on their parents that they simply refuse to face the horror of having to tell their folks."

Also in New Jersey, was the highly publicized case of Amy Grossberg, also 18, who gave birth in November 1996 in a Delaware motel. With the help of her boyfriend Brian Peterson, Jr., 19, she discarded the baby boy's body in a trash bin outside the motel. They are both charged with first degree murder. Lawyers for the two teenagers hired two forensic psychiatric experts, raising the possibility of mental illness as a defense. After the autopsy concluded the baby had been born healthy and died of multiple skull fractures and brain injuries, prosecutors indicted both Grossberg and Peterson with first-degree or intentional homicide, which is a death penalty offense. The grand jury also returned a lesser charge of first-degree murder by abuse and neglect, which carries a maximum sentence of life without parole. The second count alleges the couple recklessly caused the infant's death and engaged in an act of abuse and neglect.

While the death penalty will be a possible outcome in the Grossberg/Peterson case, according to Dr. Barbara Kirwin, a forensic psychologist, "in nearly 300 cases of women charged with neonaticide in the United States and Britain, no woman spent more than a night in jail."[52] Amy Grossberg and Brian Peterson were released on $300,000 bail each, which may indicate that the tolerance of both the legal community and our society as a whole may be reaching its limits in these types of cases. At the writing of this book, both Amy and Brian have pleaded guilty to manslaughter and Delaware has dropped its charges of murder.

In Skokie, Illinois, Cassandra Maldonado, age 17, concealed her pregnancy from everyone except two friends. She testified that she did not know that she was giving birth on November 11, 1991, and upon being startled by a noise, she let the baby's head drop into the toilet as she was being born. Cassandra did not cry out for help during labor or delivery, and her uncle and his girlfriend, who were in the house at the time, had no idea what was occurring in the bathroom. After being questioned by police, Cassandra signed a written statement which partly read, "She knew she killed [the baby]. When it was all over she said she knew if the baby was left in the water it would drown."[53] Prosecutors contended that Maldonado realized that she could not support the child and stated that she "wanted the baby to go away."

In April 1993, Cassandra was found guilty of involuntary manslaughter. Dr. Maureen Ruder, an obstetrician at Cook County Hospital, testified that Maldonado's behavior could be attributed to "extreme intimidation and pain...and a lot of pressure." The following July, Cassandra was sentenced to 1,000 hours of community service and two years of probation by Circuit Judge Joseph Romano, who said that Cassandra's real punishment "will come when she realizes the preciousness of that baby."[54]

Could this case and the others be previously depressed young women who reacted in panic with the same actions as the other mothers with postpartum depression?

ADDITIONAL RESEARCH

One recent study that appeared in the November 1997 issue of *Clinical Psychiatry News* further supports the link between a previous history of depression, mood disorders, and/or other mental problems and infanticide.[55] For the study, Dr. Margaret Spinelli, a perinatal psychiatrist and director of the maternal mental health program at the Columbia University College of Physicians and Surgeons, formally interviewed nine women being charged with murder for having allegedly committed infanticide. Her investigation included a test called the Dissociative Experiences Scale in addition to the interviews. At the interviews, Dr. Spinelli reported, the respective women "all stated somewhat the same words." Each of them described watching themselves giving birth from across the room, usually with little or no pain during delivery.

Additionally, Dr. Spinelli found that in terms of their long-term background history, each woman had been the favorite child of an overprotective, intrusive father and the rejected child of a distant, uninvolved mother. Seven of the nine women reported childhood sexual and/or physical abuse. Spinelli also reported that "...these women do not experience the symptoms of pregnancy like other women do.... Often they don't gain a lot of weight."

Spinelli's conclusion based on her findings was that a dissociative state, combined with the altered neurotransmitter levels and rapid hormone decline of the partum period can lead to "an altered mental state." Spinelli went on to state that in her opinion, these women should be treated as patients in a psychiatric ward rather than as defendants in the criminal justice system. She also pointed out that unlike the laws in the United States, British law, for example, automatically assumes that mental illness plays a role in any murder of an infant by its mother. Similarly, according to Spinelli, the results of a recent international poll revealed that 19 out of the 22 countries that responded have infanticide laws similar to British law, in which psychiatric evaluation and treatment is emphasized.

However, like any other controversial topic within the medical community, there is disagreement with Dr. Spinelli's findings amongst medical professionals. For example, forensic psychiatrist Dr. Phillip Resnick, professor of Psychiatry at Case Western Reserve Medical School in Cleveland, Ohio, disagrees, asserting that he has evaluated dozens of women who have committed infanticide and has reached a different conclusion: "In my experience, I haven't seen the history of sexual abuse. I have found that the primary motive in most women who kill their newborns is to get rid of an unwanted child. In most cases, the mother is either single or has an extramarital pregnancy."

Dissenting views like Dr. Resnick's reveal that when it comes to issues of infanticide, what causes are involved, and how these cases should be analyzed and dealt with, there is no straight, fast answer. However, the fact that Drs. Spinelli and Resnick disagree on this issue does not render either of their respective opinions useless. Perhaps both are partially correct. Certainly there are qualities which ring true in both sets of assumptions, even though Dr. Resnick questions Dr. Spinelli's data and conclusions.

The rapid decline Dr. Spinelli speaks of, and that the very dramatic change produces a psychosis and dissociative state, is certainly one of my own theories. They are not mutually exclusive. I certainly believe, along with Dr. Spinelli, that these are not 'bad' women who set about planning to kill an unwanted child.

Regardless, however of differences of opinion among the medical professionals studying these cases, the important thing is that further investigation into these areas is important in order to firmly conclude the best methods of recognizing and preventing the negative outcome. The high incidence of newborns killings highlighted in the previous section of this chapter alone should precipitate further research in this area.

GUILTY OR NOT GUILTY
BY REASON OF INSANITY?

Even as a clinician, I have found it extraordinarily difficult to define, determine, and decide whether a woman had postpartum depression or was simply cruel and amoral when she beat her child to death. Was she delusional? Was she unable, because of pathology, to control her actions? Was this learned behavior from her own background, coupled with a postpartum depression?

Rick Bragg of *The New York Times* states that "mental illness is not insanity. Depression, anxiety, and phobias are symptoms of mental illness, but not insanity. A diagnosis of insanity means that a person is delusional, schizophrenic, or psychotic." William McAninch, professor of law at the University of South Carolina, specializing in criminal and constitutional cases, elaborates on this distinction between mental illness and insanity: "The definition of guilty but mentally ill, is, in essence, [that] you know what you were doing and you knew it was wrong, but you couldn't help yourself."

In light of what we have learned about the effects of postpartum depression as a mental illness, is it not then time to revisit our view of these cases? Clearly if it not a strictly legal decision, then, we must turn to the clinicians in the women's health care field for cause, detection, and remedy.

Just as there has always been a gray area surrounding the plea of insanity, so is there a gray area surrounding infanticide.

Insanity is defined by a person's inability to know right from wrong. The clinical definition of a psychotic depression is a condition in which one's cognition is so compromised that it is impossible for the individual to grasp reality (including basic moral distinctions about what is right and what is wrong). No clinician can know for certain—post hoc—whether someone was insane at the time of the crime. However, psychotic depression or major depression with psychosis or mania are the types of syndromes that accompany postpartum crimes against children. Therefore we must consider that the mother who commits infanticide may well have a significant cognitive deficit, and we can perhaps extrapolate that she was unable to know the difference between right and wrong. I feel that these mothers should be judged as insane and receive appropriate psychiatric treatment rather than be deemed criminals who are judged within the criminal justice system and perhaps eventually sent to jail. This consideration may well apply to the following cases as well.

Take the 1994 case of Catalina Andrade who arrived severely bleeding, at Sherman Hospital in Elgin, Illinois. An emergency room physician determined that the 27-year-old-woman had just given birth, but Catalina vigorously denied this fact, and instead contended that she was a virgin and had never been pregnant.

Police, armed with a search warrant, went to her home and made a horrible discovery. Lying in the midst of garbage strewn on the basement floor, wrapped inside a plastic bag and a larger garbage bag, was the body of a newborn girl. According to Kane County Coroner Mary Lou Kearns, the baby appeared to be healthy at birth, and died of asphyxiation from the plastic bag and multiple blunt trauma to the head.[56] Catalina was charged with first-degree murder and remained under police guard for suicide. She admitted killing the infant after birth but gave no reason for the act. Family members who lived with Catalina stated that they knew nothing about the pregnancy, even though Catalina delivered a full-term, 6 1/2- to 7-pound baby girl. The baby was the fiftieth child age 14 or under to be killed in the Chicago area that year.

IN ANOTHER CASE Travia Moss thought that she was punishing little Whitney Barr for urinating on the floor. Despite being charged with first-degree murder, Travia maintains that she didn't mean to do it. However, police found evidence that there had been prior abuse of the little girl by the various healing stages of her wounds.[57]

Travia's family and friends describe her as a loving, even doting, mother who kept her children clean and well-dressed. She has two older sons, and was expecting her fourth child at the time of Whitney's death. A relative of Travia's, a cousin with four children, stated that caring for three children was probably too stressful for her.

SYLVIA VALDEZ, a mentally troubled woman, age 30, already with a history of abusing her own children, was accused in April 1996 of flinging her infant daughter from the fourth-floor window of a New York City apartment.

The baby's grandmother, Sylvia Salas, flew to Miami where Jackie, the infant, was born. Mrs. Salas promised to keep her daughter on medication and to get her psychiatric help. She rented an apartment below her own in the Bronx for the daughter. Health and Rehabilitative Services had to take the baby away from Sylvia shortly after she was born because she was neglecting her. Even before the birth the mother was talking in "dark tones" about what she might do to the baby.

Valdez refused to go to her own apartment, so she lived with her mother, Mrs. Salas who promised to watch her. One afternoon, Mrs. Salas apparently broke her promise and left her daughter alone with the baby. The baby was taking a nap when Valdez picked her up and threw her from the window. She was charged with murder.[58]

It is senseless to look back on what should have been done when the mother was obviously a mentally unbalanced women. It seems that it is still unthinkable both to the authorities who released the child to the mother and certainly to the grandmother that this could have been the result of a psychotic episode triggered by the birth of the baby.

Many possible situational as well as biological, psychological, and hormonal "triggers" may cause an episode of postpartum psychosis or debilitating mental imbalance: i.e. divorce, financial reverses, custody disputes, work or career pressures or a destructive personal relationship. As the background details and family histories in many of these cases clearly reveal, any or all of these factors may, in fact, come into play. That being the case, mental illness should not be given any less consideration as a factor/trigger than any of the other possibilities by the authorities investigating a given case.

Michael Solomon, a psychiatrist at the Northwestern University medical school, supports my assertion, saying that while directing a forensic program at the University of Virginia in recent years, he had examined many women charged with killing children. In many cases, he said, the mother was mentally ill: "I've seen several women who at other times were good, responsible caring mothers who had very severe depression with hallucinations."[59]

MUNCHAUSEN BY PROXY OR POSTPARTUM DEPRESSION?

The psychiatric nomenclature called Munchausen Syndrome is characterized by the repeated, knowing simulation of a nonexistent physical illness for the sole purpose of obtaining immediate attention and medical treatment. This disorder is well-known in psychiatric circles.

However, when cases of children displaying a wide array of medical illness began to appear in doctor's offices and hospitals, suspicion was aroused. These cases had all the earmarks of Munchausen Syndrome except that the mothers were reporting the wide array of symptoms not about themselves, but about their children.

I'm sure a great many cases that fell into this category simply went by unnoticed by doctors, as they got busy taking care of whatever the symptom the child had. In these instances, the mother would always be well-informed about medical terms and syndromes. The degree of her knowledge and sophistication about various illnesses would make it difficult for the physician to detect the false nature of the child's illness. These mothers would then support the history and symptoms they gave regarding the child by tampering with diagnostic procedures. For example, they would find ways to change body temperature in the child, either by manipulation or substitution of a thermometer. They would contaminate urine samples with feces, blood, or saliva in order to suggest infection or other illnesses.

All these characteristics were concomitant with Munchausen Syndrome, except that the patient was a child and the reporter was the mother.

In one recent case, Mary Bryk, a 38-year-old nurse, wrote a shocking article on this topic, relating how her mother's abuse of her as a child resulted in eight years of needless hospitalizations and surgical procedures.

She wrote of the permanent scars that were the result of her mother slamming her ankle with a hammer when she was two, and of how her feet ended up being different shoe sizes. Then her mother would intentionally infect her open wounds with coffee grounds and dirt. She claimed that the abuse was aimed at getting attention for her mother.

In response to cases like this one, the new nomenclature was born—Munchausen Syndrome By Proxy. Experts called it 'a psychological disorder' in which parents make their children sick—or just pretend their children are sick—so they can gain attention and appear as saviors, regardless of the effect on the children.

In 1992, a Florida woman was accused of making her baby daughter sick in an attempt to get attention and may have done the same thing to her infant son who had died two years before. According to doctors, Christina Rubio suffers from Munchausen Syndrome By Proxy.

This case began in May 1990, when Christina's 13-month-old son P.J. died from an illness that baffled doctors. Thirteen months after his death, P.J.'s sister Lauren was born, and she began to show the same symptoms of whatever killed P.J. A police search of Lauren's hospital room yielded three bottles of a medication, Ipecac, used to induce vomiting, found in her mother's pocketbook, a chemical which was also found in P.J.'s preserved organs. Too much of the drug can cause heart failure.

Little P.J. died less than a month after he was treated for a stomach disorder. He died of "vascular myopathy of cardiac and skeletal muscles"—damaged by the Ipecac, which can damage heart, skeletal and other muscles if taken chronically.

Dr. Deborah Day, an Orlando psychologist who is preparing a book on the syndrome and was treating seven cases stated: "In hospitals, the mothers are there all the time. The staff makes comments about how wonderful they are. Munchausen Syndrome [By Proxy] is the most misunderstood form of child abuse we've seen."

Christina Rubio was arrested, after which Orlando police alerted the St. Petersburg police of P.J.'s death, initiating a full investigation. Christina was sentenced to 13 years in prison for killing her son, to be followed by 20 years of probation.[60]

There is still a great deal of disagreement regarding the basis for Munchausen Syndrome. Many feel that an atypical depression may well be the basis for the bizarre behavior of these mothers. If so, there certainly would need a reexamination on what part may be a postpartum depression as well as a bearing on Munchausen Syndrome By Proxy.

INTERNATIONAL HEADLINE CASES

It is important to remember that cases of women's depression and the subsequent behaviors involving their families is not exclusive to the United States. There are reports of similar cases all over the world. Of course, we are usually not able to be informed of the propensity of this problem.

The report from a French medical journal by F. Desseigne and J. Carrere, cited previously in Chapter Two, did not address itself to the medical and legal aspects of the problem, but rather to the origin of the behaviors as connected to their social, affective, and sexual components.

Of course when there is a dangerous patient who has been hospitalized, the facts may come to light. A cursory examination of the archives at the Henri-Colin facility uncovered the discovery of more than 12 cases.

Let's compare a few of these with some of our own well-known cases. The authors write that in general those women belong to a very modest social class, their family environment was bad, and their marriages were often their escape from restrictive or even abusive families.

One of the women described came from a broken family in which her father left her mother when she was 16 months old. Her mother had been a teenager when she became pregnant and had to marry the father.

The woman exhibited a relatively high intellect, attended school until she was 16, and then took secretarial classes. Her first pregnancy interrupted her professional activity, but she returned to work just after the baby's birth. Four months after the birth of this first child, she became pregnant with her second. She stated that that is when she became "bad."

The woman turned against her husband and could not bear to look at him and became "frigid" after the second child. She also turned against her neighbors. She began to have conflicts regarding the new baby.

The husband had had an unhappy childhood, but nevertheless seemed like a nice, simple, rather intelligent albeit immature individual. He was very jealous, and said he never cheated on his wife.

Their housing conditions were poor, with only one bedroom, that included the children's beds along with the couple's. There was no water or heat.

In October 1969, the husband returned from work and found his wife, prostrate, covered with blood. Her two children were dead in their beds, the four year old killed by strangulation and the three year old by a fractured skull.

During the investigation, she stated the "her husband wanted to leave her and take the children with him." When she spoke of the "accident," she said only, "I cannot have been so wild, there must have been somebody else in the house." In addition, she didn't understand or remember any object she might have used to kill the children.

Her history reports that since the age of 19, she suffered from migraine headaches that included loss of consciousness. The headaches were associated with a state of "sadness" during her menstruation. In 1967, she fell into a depressive state and attempted suicide with an overdose of medication. She was hospitalized at La Pitie's hospital in Paris.

She described her depressive state as being "shut down and plagued with frequent bloody dreams." She read detective stories while her mother took care of her household. She stated that she wanted to die with her children. She did not want any other woman to touch her children. Talking about her mother, she said, "She will not have them."

The rest of the subsequent psychiatric report read as follows:

❧ "Serious and acute reactionary depressive state without melancholia. Emotional instability with hyper-emotional neurosis. Migraine syndrome. Biological factors. Crime committed during menstruation. She still represents a danger to herself because of the persistence of a depressive mood. Very fragile personality subject to impulses. Probably psychotic nucleus."

❧ When hospitalized, the certificate stated: "Acute psychopathic state. A few scars seem to evoke previous suicidal attempts."

❧ Fifteen days later, the certificate states: "Psycho-neurotic depressive syndrome with important frustration and inhibition and annihilation behaviors which led to the committing of a double murder of her children."

❧ Placement request: "To take advantage of permissions under the control of her husband in order to establish a social reinsertion".

❧ Currently: "The patient left Henri-Colin section. The husband found another apartment with all the 'utilities.' She resumed her former career and has been working regularly since then. Married life seems good. Would the past be erased?"

Without continuing to describe the 15 cases, my perusal of the French research articles reveal that almost all the cases have history of one or more suicidal attempts or ideation. However, it is only at the conclusion and after more recent examination of the 15 cases that some of the cases are thought to be postpartum depression.

A prevailing characteristic of many of the mothers is their expression of the desire to prevent the children from the suffering associated with existence.

In only one of 15 cases in France did the original psychiatrist say, "The symptomatic stupor state brought by a postpartum psychosis was already present during the delivery but remained unnoticed due to the woman's ignorance of the French language." The woman in question in this case was of Algerian nationality.

The authors point out that "transplantation into a metropolitan area like Paris, a pregnancy, the birth of a child always create problems on a subject who is already fragile, poorly structured, and unable to face responsibilities. The arrival of a child can very well provoke new manifestations of anxiety with a person who formerly showed states of melancholic depression."

"Such facts reveal one thing: the [current] medical attitude needs to be questioned when it comes to the depressive state of pregnant women, whether depression occurs prior to or during the pregnancy. It is a fact that... medical examinations [in France] are too quick and do not investigate the psychiatric past of the patient well enough to identify depressive antecedents. Prevention of those behaviors could be conducted with a closer look to a prior history of psycho-affectivity or psycho-social difficulties."[61]

It is this same sentiment that I would like to bring to bear on the similar cases that have taken place in the United States, those cited in this book as well as others that we hear about only after the fact, when the tragedy has already occurred. The cases described above are particularly painful in light of how similar it sounds to many of the other cases examined in this book. The point is simple. Postpartum depression and progressive postpartum depression can—and docs—affect women all over the world. Since this condition inevitably affects the families of these women, it essentially is a problem that concerns everyone. And in most cases, its signs appear long before an act of violence occurs. Therefore, the best strategy to take is preventative. We must establish better support systems in which these signs can be recognized *before* they result in tragedy, rather than after.

Darlie Routier, whose case was described earlier in this chapter, was sentenced to die for her crime by lethal injection. Seven woman, and five men passed down this extremely rare sentence. According to the Death Penalty Information Center, Washington, only five other women in the country are on death row for killing their children.

Darlie showed no visible emotion as the verdict was read. Apparently the jury felt that she presented a continuing threat to society and that there were no mitigating circumstances that might make a life prison sentence a more appropriate punishment.

George Kendall, staff counsel with the Capital Punishment Project at the NAACP Legal Defense and Education Fund, said the jury's sentence was unusual because society usually does not tend to think of women who kill their children as habitual criminals, but rather as people beset by mental troubles.

But Bryan Stevenson, director of the Equal Justice Initiative, an organization based in Alabama that provides legal assistance to capital defendants said, "It used to be that when these crimes took place, the feeling was less that this was criminal than that this was tragic."[62]

The point that I'd like to make with regard to these shifting views on the behaviors that sometimes result from untreated PPD and PPPD is that the one thing that has been constant throughout the ages is the attitude of either dismissiveness, neglect, ignorance, denial, or all of the above, by family members, doctors, counselors, friends, clergy, and even the mother herself. These postpartum ill-nesses have usually not been taken seriously unless the condition has worsened considerably to such an extent that a tragedy occurs. Emphasis has been placed on interpreting the tragic outcomes rather than their underlying causes. The fact is that preventive treatment—which, thankfully, in this day and age *is* available—has not been the focus. And it should be.

Like the other cases I have described, the cases which have made headline news illustrate the relationship of progressive postpartum depression to mood disorders and how the birth of a child produces a trigger that in some people result in a lifetime of misery.

As Dr. Mark Gold wrote in 1986 in his book, *The Good News About Depression:*

"Despite the high incidence of depression following childbirth, the often desperate new mother may receive inappropriate or inade-quate treatment—or, most likely, no treatment at all. Psychiatrists, notes a commentator in the *Journal of American Medical Association,* are not taught to differentiate these mood disorders from those not related to childbirth; 'psychiatry training programs and texts refuse to separate them from non-postpartum conditions, or recognize them as distinct disorders.'"[63]

Sadly, the situation has not significantly changed and the head-line cases continue to appear. Depressive disorders, or mood disor-ders, sometimes the lifetime result of the postpartum trigger, can easily be treated by modern medicine. When untreated, the disorder progresses and carries its effects from generation to generation. But once the mother and clinicians are informed, the severity of its effects can be ameliorated as can the effects of many other genetic illness.

7 | GETTING HELP

RECENTLY, WHILE 'SURFING the Net,' I came across an article about pregnancy in the *Family Planet News*. It was entitled "New Baby Blues," and was dated Monday, May 13, 1996. "Good," I thought, "someone is trying to inform and hopefully prevent another expectant mother of the possible danger of postpartum depression."

Actually, it turned out to be a good article by The American College of Obstetricians and Gynecologists. I decided to include a reprint in *A Mother's Tears*, since I feel anything positive and informative is important. The article referred to a free pamphlet with even more information on postpartum depression. Here's the article itself:

"SOON AFTER GIVING birth, a majority of mothers (about 70 percent) experience mood swings in some form—crying spells, sleeplessness, loss of appetite, irritability, anger, or an inability to make decisions. These feelings are know as the 'baby blues,' and they pass quickly within a few days or a week. They are a natural reaction to physical, hormonal, and psychological changes.

"About ten percent of mothers experience intense anxiety or hopelessness that lingers for longer than two weeks or which surfaces a month or two after childbirth. This is a more serious problem known as postpartum depression. Other signals include sleeplessness, even when tired; sleeping too much; changes in appetite; worrying excessively about your baby or family or, conversely, feeling unconcerned; panic attacks; or fears that you might harm the baby or yourself. These feelings may come regardless of age or whether you have previously given birth. As with other types of depression, the precise cause may be difficult to pin down. Your mood may be hormonally induced, and you also may be overwhelmed by life circumstances and stressful events. Researchers have found that after giving birth, levels of a hormone that helps mediate body temperature, appetite, and sleep tend to be suppressed. Over extended periods, this may contribute to mood disturbances.

"Women who lack a supportive spouse or family also face an increased risk of postpartum depression. Women who have recently gone through a stressful event such as the loss of a loved one, a family illness, or a move to another city are another at-risk group. If you have a previous history of depression or other emotional difficulties, you may be vulnerable.

"If you suspect you have a postpartum depression, talk to your doctor or ask for a referral to a mental-health specialist. There are effective ways to treat this condition. Counseling or drug treatment, or a combination of the two, may be recommended. Some medications are safe to use even if you are breast-feeding, but check with your doctor. Joining a support group may also help.

"If you don't seek help for your depression, it may go on indefinitely, making you less able to cope with your family and work responsibilities. Support will help you feel and function better during this special time in your life.

"For a free copy of a pamphlet 'Postpartum Depression,' send a stamped, self-addressed, business-size envelope to the American College of Obstetricians and Gynecologists, Resource Center/APO91, 409 12th Street, SW, P.O. Box 96920, Washington, D.C. 20090-6920."[64]

Finally, I also wanted to leave readers with a list of resources that would help them know where to go to for further information on postpartum depression and related issues. Iylene Barsky's own experiences coupled with her keen clinical sense of detection, treatment, and resources make her uniquely qualified to put together the resource guide that follows and forms the bulk of this chapter.

GETTING HELP
by Ilyene Barsky, LCSW

It is important to note that there are very distinct markers which are easy to read in advance in the cases of these depressions and treatments are available. This book is designed to be a primer on the subject and can clearly elucidate the resources which are available. Dr. Huysman has written a comprehensive text on the Who, What, and When that postpartum depression encompasses.

It is not unusual for a woman seeking help for postpartum depression to be confronted with health care professionals who know little about the illness, research, or treatment. Like many other women, I was helped in spite of this lack of expertise. It was not until years later, after the birth of my second child, that I finally understood what happened to me.

Like most new mothers, I had certain expectations of what motherhood would be like. My first child was conceived immediately. Very planned. Very wanted. My husband and I, both mental health professionals in our mid-twenties had promising careers and a hard-earned down payment on our first new home. Life was good.

Then through a series of events, construction on our home was delayed. The year was 1980. We watched helplessly as our mortgage interest rate soared from 9 percent to 14 percent. Regardless, I took maternity leave one month prior to my due date and one week later, we moved into our new home. That same night, amidst cartons and unassembled baby furniture, I went into labor. Gavin was born April 20, 1980—three and one-half weeks premature, weighing in at 4 pounds, 8 ounces, and jaundiced. He remained in the hospital for two additional days after I was discharged. On day eight, he was down to four pounds, still a little jaundiced, but stable and healthy enough to take home. This is where my nightmare began.

The onset of what would become a severe, classical case of postpartum depression was insidious. The stage was set: financial problems, isolation, loss of job, lack of social support, and a premature, "colicky" baby.

Restless nights gave way to chronic insomnia. Fatigue gave way to severe exhaustion and lethargy. "Normal" feelings of insecurity that go along with being a new mother gave way to a total collapse of self-esteem and an inability to cope with day to day activities. I seldom showered, washed my hair, or brushed my teeth. I wore the same housedress every day. I did not care.

But the most disturbing, frightening symptoms of all were the obsessions. They were the horribly vivid, repetitive thoughts of something catastrophic happening to my son and/or to myself. I knew the thoughts were irrational ("ego alien"), but they would not go away. If I was able to catch any sleep, I was jolted into wakefulness as those images permeated my dreams.

I searched my psychology and social work textbooks for an explanation, a "cure," an answer, anything. I looked in books on crisis intervention. I looked in books on parenthood. Nothing. I knew I was in trouble. Finally, after nine months of suffering, withdrawal and spiraling despair, I sought the help of a psychiatrist.

I was diagnosed with "Major Depression" and placed on antidepressant medication. Within days I was able to sleep and other symptoms slowly began to subside. Follow-up consisted of "medication management." Period.

EARLY DETECTION IS CRUCIAL

To this day, I am asked, "How did you go on that long without being noticed?"

Easy—I hid it. Close friends and family chalked it up to my being "moody" or "sensitive." I avoided going out and forming new relationships. My husband did urge me to see a doctor, but was himself emotionally "unavailable." Perhaps he was experiencing his own PPD (minus the hormone imbalance), which, by the way, is *not uncommon* for new fathers.

But a more important question than 'how did I go on that long?' is *why* did I go that long? The answer is that like most women struggling with PPD, I was ashamed and embarrassed. I had bought into the myth of maternal bliss, believed my feelings were invalid, and that there was something innately wrong with me. I felt inadequate and guilt-ridden. I kept hoping "it," which had taken on a life of its own, would just go away by itself and no one would ever have to know. And, or course, the longer I waited, the worse "it" got.

Over the years, I have seen the scenario played out with my own PPD patients. Their resistance to seeking treatment is reinforced by their own lack of knowledge and our society's expectations of new mothers. And in spite of developments in the last ten to fifteen years, there are still those professionals who deny or minimize the existence of this biological and psychosocial disorder. My heart goes out to those women whose health care providers invalidates her feelings and actually pushes her into a deeper state of distress.

One patient told me that after two months of depression and severe anxiety, she finally reached out to her obstetrician. He told her to "buy a red sweater and have her husband take her out to dinner." I wish I had a dime for each time a woman was told by her health care professional that this condition is "normal." "Don't worry about it." "It will go away."

This lack of information on the part of the professional community, the postpartum woman, and our society as a whole has all to often led to tragic consequences.

WHERE TO START?

My daughter, Monica, was born by emergency Caesarean Section 3 1/2 years later. Though delighted to have a daughter, I was disappointed at having to deliver her by "C-Section." The crying, at the time inexplicable, began two days later. When my primary obstetrician came to my hospital room to examine me, I told him that whenever his associate (who delivered my baby) came into my room, I would start crying.

He laughed and told me his associate had the same effect on him, jotted some notes in my chart, and left the room. There was also an incident involving a "floating" nurse who came to my room to "help" me during the first postpartum night. She clearly did not want to be in the obstetrics unit with private patients and made a point of telling me so. Still I needed help getting to the bathroom, as I was drugged and still unable to support myself. She told me, "Women like you have it too easy and need to do for yourself." She proceeded to tell me that she usually worked in the wards with indigent patients and reluctantly got me to the bathroom. I reported her the next day, but never learned the outcome.

These two incidents so deeply affected me that once home, I contacted my Lamaze instructor. (She had given our class her telephone number and asked us to call her if we had any problems after the delivery.) I was depressed and weepy but in no way despondent as I was after my first pregnancy. I was still on anti-depressant medication. Lorrie Thomas, my instructor, was wonderful. She listened sympathetically, offered support, and validated my feelings. She even asked me to write an article for the local Childbirth Education Association's (CEA) newsletter. I wanted to do this "right" and did a little research on childbirth experiences. And then I found it… a little article in a magazine describing symptoms of postpartum depression. I could not believe it. This "thing" I had after my first child was born had a name. I was not alone.

I now had "permission" to discuss my postpartum experience. I wrote my article and was invited to speak at the next CEA meeting. To my amazement, two of the instructors shared (for the first time) their experiences with PPD. I was encouraged to spread the word. I spoke at other instructors meetings and was urged to educate the public.

By 1985, I was armed with facts, figures, and research, and became a guest speaker for special interest groups like La Leche League and "Mothers of Twins." Women with PPD began to trickle into my office. In 1986 I gave birth to my third "child," The Center for Postpartum Adjustment.

I've loved, nurtured, and watched her grow. In the last 13 years, I have treated hundreds of PPD sufferers and have become a regular speaker at hospitals and birth center. I present seminars to those professionals who serve as the front-line people to those women in the grips of a postpartum illness. Issues such as risk factor and early detection are addressed. They *are* listening and have become the primary referral sources for those women who are suffering.

- ✦ OB/GYNs and Midwives—These are the professionals who have cared for the woman up until the time of delivery and follow-up. They are the first line of defense. Their sensitivity to and awareness of postpartum disorders is critical.

- ✦ Pediatricians—An observant pediatrician will note not only the progress of the newborn, but the adjustment of the new mother as well.

- ✦ Hospitals and Birth Centers—OB nurses and the Offices of Community Education should be able to direct the postpartum sufferer to an appropriate resource.

- ✦ Childbirth Educators—More and more instructors are incorporating a lecture on postpartum disorders into their curriculum. Dads especially need to pay attention as the expectant mother usually denies that it will ever happen to her.

- ✦ La Leche Groups and Lactation Consultants—If well-informed, these resources will know that a nursing mother is most vulnerable to a postpartum episode when she weans her baby and experiences another hormone drop.

- ✦ Doula Services—These organizations provide the new mother with physical and emotional support during the "fourth trimester." A *doula* helps with the shopping, cooking, and other domestic chores. She is there to free up the new mother to settle in with her new family and to help with the baby so the mother can relax. She is also there to suggest outside help if she observes anything out of the ordinary.

➤ Non-Profit Community Organizations—These organizations, such as Planned Parenthood and The Mental Health Association, should be able to recommend a postpartum specialist. Local organizations such as Mommy and Me, Caesarean Support Groups, and Mothers of Twins and Triplets can be found in neighborhood newspapers or through doctors offices. They, too, may provide a link between the postpartum woman and a mental health professional.

MENTAL HEALTH PROFESSIONALS

Ideally, the best form of treatment would be a team approach, addressing the biological, psychological, and social aspects of postpartum disorders. These professionals may work in conjunction with one another or might become involved at different stages of treatment.

The woman seeking their services must remember that she is a consumer and when selecting psychotherapist, has the right to ask questions about his/her practice, philosophy, educational background and experience in working with PPD. For example, not all therapists are aware that postpartum disorders can manifest themselves as anxiety, panic attacks, and obsessive-compulsive disorders. Misdiagnosis and the wrong treatment can be damaging.

The complaints I hear most frequently about psychotherapists are:

➤ "He/She did not listen to me—he/she just gave me drugs."
➤ "He/She was looking for something deep-seated like my relationship with my mother. My mother and I love each other and don't have any 'unresolved conflicts.'"
➤ "He/She did not say anything. There was no feedback."

Unfortunately, even at the professional level, lack of knowledge does exist. If a woman is not connecting with her therapist, she needs to find another. This is extremely difficult when she is feeling so vulnerable. Access to *qualified* care and interventions rests largely with an appropriate referral made by Local Resources and/or National/International Organizations (listed in this chapter).

Psychotherapists vary in their credentials, training, style, and individual personalities. However, at the very least, they should be objective, supportive, and non-judgmental. Those most commonly involved in the treatment of postpartum disorders include the following:

➤ Psychiatrists—Psychiatrists are licensed physicians (M.D. or D.O.) that have additional training in emotional and biological mental illnesses. They generally use medication as the primary mode of treatment, although some practice psychotherapy as well. If not, they can refer a patient to another discipline who can. These are the only therapists who can write prescriptions.

➤ Clinical Psychologists—Clinical psychologists should have a doctoral degree (Ph.D. or Psy.D.) and have passed a certifying exam in order to be licensed by their state. They can administer and interpret psychological test and have specialized training in psychotherapy. They can recommend medications and often work in consultation with a psychiatrist.

➤ Clinical Social Workers—Social workers should have a master's (MSW) or doctoral (DSW, Ph.D.) degree and should also be licensed by their state (LSW, LCSW). They have considerable training and experience in practicing psychotherapy. They can make referrals to psychiatrists if medication is needed.

➤ Marriage and Family Counselors—Family counselors have a minimum of a master's degree and generally work with people in the context of relationships and family systems rather than individual issues.

❥ Psychiatric Nurses (R.N.s)—Psychiatric R.N.s, as this nickname indicates, have a degree in nursing from university. They may have a bachelor's degree, master's degree, or Ph.D.s. They usually work with a psychiatrist and can provide counseling and psychotherapy. If they have advanced ARNP credentials, they are working in conjunction with a doctor.

❥ Pastoral Counselors—These counselors are ordained clergy persons who focus on religious issues in therapy.

NATIONAL / INTERNATIONAL ORGANIZATIONS

By the mid 1980s a quiet revolution was brewing. Women were talking and sharing their postpartum experiences. Support groups were forming locally, nationally, and internationally. It was through a patient in 1986 that I learned about Depression After Delivery (D.A.D.) has become the cornerstone for groups and organizations that now stretch across the United States.

Now, women suffering with PPD can have direct lines to sharing, support, and information all over the world.

DEPRESSION AFTER DELIVERY (D.A.D.)
P.O. Box 1282, Morrisville, PA 19067
Telephone: (800) 944-4773

Depression After Delivery (D.A.D.) is a national non-profit organization staffed by volunteers. Founded in Trenton, New Jersey in 1985, it was the first group of its kind in the United States. Its founder, Nancy Berchtold, organized the group following her own experience with postpartum psychosis. D.A.D. provides support, education, information and referrals to women undergoing postpartum distress. A quarterly newsletter, "Heart Strings," is included with membership.

POSTPARTUM SUPPORT INTERNATIONAL (PSI)
927 North Kellogg Avenue, Santa Barbara, CA 93111
Telephone: (805) 967-7636

Postpartum Support International (PSI) founded by Jane Honikman in 1987, is a worldwide network which focuses on pre- and postpartum mental health and social support. Their goal is to provide treatment for postpartum depression, psychosis, and anxiety disorders. Members have access to their lending library which includes books, articles, videos, audio tapes, and slides. PSI encourages formation of new support groups, the strengthening of existing groups and addresses, and legal and insurance coverage issues. PSI serves as a link for women seeking help elsewhere in the country and sponsors an annual conference to review its progress in achieving their goals. Its founder has also undertaken the arduous task of forming a Pen Pal Program for women who are incarcerated as the result of a crime precipitated by a postpartum illness.

PACIFIC POSTPARTUM SUPPORT SOCIETY (PPPSS)
Suite 104—1416 Commercial Drive, Vancouver, BC
Canada V5L3X9
Telephone: (604) 255-7999

Pacific Postpartum Support Society (PPPSS) offers telephone support, support groups, training, and written information worldwide. Their book, *Postpartum Depression and Anxiety—A Self-Help Guide for Mothers,* revised for the third edition, has sold of 13,000 copies to date. PPPSS is the oldest self-help group dealing with postpartum disorders, having been founded over 20 years ago.

MARCE' SOCIETY
North American Representative: Michael O'Hara, Ph.D.
Department of Psychology
University of Iowa, Iowa City, IA 52242
Telephone: (319) 335-2452

The Marce' Society was founded in England in 1980. It is named for Dr. Louis Victor Marce, who published a comprehensive study of postpartum psychosis in France in 1858. He identified postpartum psychiatric disorders as a physical illness. Today, the society is committed to improving the understanding, treatment, and prevention of postpartum disorders. The society also sponsors an annual international conference.

WOMEN'S HEALTH CONNECTION
P.O. Box 6338, Madison, WI 53716-0338
Telephone: (800) 266-6632

Women's Health Connection is the educational division of Women's International Pharmacy. Their newsletter, "Connections," is dedicated to the education and management of hormone related disorders. They can connect women with pharmaceutical sources for obtaining natural progesterone and estrogen.

ICEA
P.O. Box 20048, Minneapolis, MN 55420
Telephone: (800) 624-4934
International Childbirth Education Association (ICEA) is an interdisciplinary organization representing groups and individuals, parent and professional, who share an interest in family-centered maternity care.

BOOKS AND VIDEOS

We've come a long way since 1980 when I searched through text-books in the hopes of understanding what was happening to me. PPD is not a new phenomenon. Hippocrates recognized and described the condition centuries ago. However, between the 1920s and 1980, it was widely believed that postpartum disorders were not different that any other psychiatric problem. Hence, little was written and little was taught. Because postpartum disorders lie somewhere between obstetrics and psychiatry, it fell between the cracks and received little attention from either discipline. Today, most experts agree that there is a physical link between the mind and that postpartum disorders need to be approached from the biological, social, and psychological fields.

The following books reflect current research and are the ones I most often recommend to my patients.

Belsky, Jan and John Kelly, *Transition to Parenthood: How a First Child Changes a Marriage.* New York: Delacorte Press, 1994.— Based on the findings of the Penn State Child and Family Development Project.

Blumfield, Wendy, *Life After Birth: Every Woman's Guide to the First Year of Motherhood.* Great Britain: Element Books, 1992.—Addresses fantasy vs. the reality of pregnancy and birth, learning and adapting to new routines, and identity changes for mother and father.

Comport, Maggie, *Surviving Motherhood: Coping with Postnatal Depression.* Great Britain: Ashgrove Press, 1990.—Offers advice on how to look at the experience of postpartum depression as an opportunity for growth.

Dalton, Katarina, *Depression After Childbirth*. Great Britain: Oxford University Press, 1980.—One of PPD's pioneers tells how to recognize and treat postpartum illness. Emphasis on hormonal aspects of this disorder.

Dix, Carol, *The New Mother Syndrome: Coping with Postpartum Stress and Depression*. New York: Pocket Books, 1985.—This is *the book* that brought PPD out of the closet and into the public's attention. Difficult to find. Can be ordered through Depression After Delivery, also known as D.A.D. (see National Resources).

Dunnewald, Ann and Diane Sanford, *The Postpartum Survival Guide*. California: New Harbinger Publications, 1994.—Covers the entire spectrum of postpartum adjustment problems. Includes biological, psychological, and psychosocial risk factors; symptom management, prevention, and recovery. Special attention is given to single, older, and adoptive mothers.

Hamilton, James Alexander and Patricia Neel Harberger, *Postpartum Psychiatric Illness: A Picture Puzzle*. Philadelphia: University of Pennsylvania Press, 1992.—Written by one of the leading authorities in the field of postpartum disorders. This clinical study is geared toward both the professional and layperson. Author's Note: A must for the more informed reader. This is the *best* resource available on this subject, but unfortunately does not appear on the shelves of bookstores under what expectant mothers should know; available in libraries on request.

Hotchner, Tracy, *Childbirth and Marriage: The Transition to Parenthood*. New York: Avon Books, 1988.—Guide for new parents confronting the challenge of balancing their relationship with the tasks of child rearing. Promotes trust in parental instincts.

Kitzinger, Sheila, *The Year After Childbirth*. Toronto: HarperCollins, 1994.—This compassionate and comprehensive guide with over 300 pictures and drawings, provides practical advice and support for this turbulent year.

Kleiman, Karen, and Valerie Raskin, *This Isn't What I Expected: Recognizing and Recovering from Depression and Anxiety After Childbirth*. New York: Bantam, 1994.—Contains information on treatment options (medications, psychotherapy, ECT); how to deal with panic-attacks, obsessive-compulsive urges, and postpartum emergencies; and the loss of self-esteem associated with motherhood complicated by PPD.

Misiri, Shaila, *Shouldn't I Be Happy?: Emotional Problems of Pregnant and Postpartum Women*. New York: Free Press, 1995.—Addresses anxiety and depression during the pre- and postpartum periods, as well as issues surrounding breast-feeding and eating disorders during pregnancy.

Pacific Postpartum Support Society, *Postpartum Depression and Anxiety: A Self-Help Guide for Mothers*. Vancouver, BC, Canada: Grandview Printing Co., 1987.—A practical book based on the experiences of thousands of thousands of women and what helped them get through this time. Order direct from Pacific Postpartum Support Society (See International Resources).

Placksin, Sally, *Mothering the New Mother*. New York: Newmarket Press, 1994.—Based on the research and personal experience of the author. Filled with practical suggestions, listings of newsletters, books, hotlines, video cassettes, and support groups.

Price, Jane, *Motherhood: What It Does to Your Mind*. London: Pandora Press, 1988.—Addresses the emotional aspects of motherhood during every stage from the decision to conceive to the postpartum period. Examines myths and pressures of mothering as imposed by society.

Sapstead, Anne Marie, *Banish Post-Baby Blues.* Great Britain: Thorsons Publishing Group, 1990.—Contains anecdotes, facts, figures, definitions, and encouragement. Special attention paid to actual birth experiences and to fathers.

VIDEOS

Fragile Beginnings: Postpartum Mood and Anxiety Disorders
Lifecycle Productions, 1993.
Telephone: (617) 964-0047

Hope and Healing Postpartum Depression
Vancouver, Canada: British Columbia Reproductive Care Program, 1993.
Telephone: (604) 255-7999

You're Not Alone
Vancouver, Canada: Pacific Postpartum Support Society
Telephone: (604) 255-7999

Postpartum Emotions: The Blues and Beyond
Austin, Texas: Family Experiences Productions, 1995.
Telephone: (512) 338-1318

ILYENE BARSKY is a licensed clinical social worker who has practiced psychiatric and medical social work since 1977. She received her master's degree from Barry University and is a member of the

Academy of Certified Social Workers and the National Association of Social Workers.

Ms. Barsky has specialized in the treatment of postpartum disorders since 1984, following her own experience with PPD. An advocate for sufferers of PPD who works closely with Depression After Delivery and Postpartum Support International, she has presented regular seminars for professionals and the lay public, appeared on several local television shows, and written nationally syndicated articles on PPD.

Ms. Barsky is a single parent who resides in Davie, Florida with her two teenagers. Her practice is called The Center for Postpartum Adjustment, 1515 North University Drive, Suite 116A, Coral Springs, Florida 33071, Telephone: (954) 752-0460, Fax: (954) 752-4542.

EPILOGUE

NO ONE WANTS to think about the dark side of the early days of motherhood. Before PPD and PPPD were identified as recognizable, treatable mood disorders, it could have been argued that there was little use in focusing on the existence of these conditions since we knew so little about what, if anything, could be done to treat and prevent them. This, however, is no longer the case.

Today, anyone with access to a medical community that is aware that PPD is a serious and fairly common problem, a television, and books can potentially get treatment if they need it before a tragedy ensues. Nevertheless, many doctors are unaware of the frequency and severity of postpartum illnesses, as are most women, and the type of media coverage these type of disorders get still focuses on the tragic products of the disease rather than its prevention. So the long and short of it is that we still have a long way to go.

Invaluable resources and information on postpartum illnesses that did not exist at all 20 to 30 years ago are now available. We don't have all the answers, but we know a great deal more helpful information than we once did. Now, we need to spread the word so it can be properly utilized.

As is the case with many illnesses that have potentially terrifying consequences, with regard to postpartum depression, most people want to believe that it is rare and therefore that 'it could never happen to me.' Nevertheless, as the frightening statistics indicate, the reality is that these people are wrong. At least five children a day die from abuse and neglect around this country, more that 2000 every year.[65] In Florida, where I practice, there were 63 deaths in 1995 alone. Ninety percent of the cases nationwide involved children under the age of one year. As stated previously in Chapter 6, the Federal Bureau of Investigation's most recent statistics indicate that approximately five infants under the age of one are killed in the U.S. every week, an estimate based on data gathered in 1995. Similarly, according to FBI records, 662 children under the age of five were murdered in 1992. Ernest Allen, president of the National Center for missing and exploited children, estimates that about two-thirds of those victims were killed by one or both of their parents.

On a similar note, one follow-up study of postpartum illness reflected that if a depressive disorder began at postpartum, the probability of a recurrent affective disorder was 43 percent for unipolar depression and 66 percent for bipolar disorder. The risk of developing another postpartum illness varied from one in three to one in five pregnancies. Five percent of the sample ultimately committed suicide, and the probable incidence of infanticide was four percent.[66] In other words, women with postpartum depression often had recurrences with as many as one in twenty leading to suicide or the killing of a child.

Finally, according to *The Harvard Mental Health Letter,* "about 15 percent of new mothers' (symptoms) deepen into a more serious and lasting postpartum depression." The report further states that one out of l,000 new mothers has a psychotic episode, usually in the first few weeks.[67]

My aim in citing these statistics is not to simply scold the medical community, or to merely scare expectant mothers or their families, but rather to incite them all to act: by educating themselves on the existence and nature of this illness. Whether one is a doctor, an expectant mother, or a concerned family member or friend, being well-informed is the best way to catch a potentially disastrous case of PPD early on and prevent a woman from harming her children, her partner, and/or herself. The extreme, tragic cases cited throughout this book—cases like those involving Susan Smith, whose family background was fraught for years with depression, suicide, and turmoil— prompt a closer look at the professionals who could have helped the women involved, as well as family and friends who could have identified the ominous signs. Women and their significant others in particular need to be aware—for forewarned is forearmed.

The writing of this book has been both a labor of love and a monumental task. Every time I examined a case, investigating clues for diagnosis and recording the information, I felt pain for both the mothers and the children.

Even condensing the reports journalistically eventually did not reduce my feelings of pain. I came to realize that working with one woman, one case at a time, was one thing. But having to touch so many tragedies, *knowing they could have been avoided,* was altogether different. The hardest part of all was recording the words of the mothers in personal interviews and seeing firsthand the impact on the event that will remain with them for the rest of their lives. I found myself crying for the innocent children who loved and trusted their mothers. I also cried for the mothers who grew into unrecognizable personalities, unable to control the illness which overcame them.

As each case appeared in the headlines, the community, wherever it was, reacted with horror. Then, somehow, after the mourning, the grief, the shock, the memory of the horror dissolved.

However, these memories remain with me. They have left me with new resolve to inform, educate, and attempt to intervene whenever and wherever possible. I hope you will all join me in this educational crusade.

BIBLIOGRAPHY

IN DOING THE RESEARCH for *A Mother's Tears,* I have utilized many articles and reports from the writers of the *Miami Herald, The Wichita Eagle, The Chicago Tribune, The New York Times, Time, Newsweek,* and many other fine newspapers, periodicals, and magazines. I would like to express my admiration and gratitude to the journalists—particularly those on the crime beat—whose meticulous work enabled me to delve more deeply into the issues and circumstances surrounding postpartum depression and the sometimes disastrous consequences of untreated cases.

The most important and frequently used of those periodical sources are listed in the bibliography below along with the books I consulted. For additional reference information on the other articles from periodicals and newspapers, please see endnotes.

Beck, C.T., "The Lived Experience of Postpartum Depression: A Phenomenological Study," *Nurs. Res* 41 (3), 1992: 188-170.
Berger, Diane & Lisa, *We Heard the Angels of Madness.* New York: Quill William Morrow, 1991.

Burak, Carl S., & Michele G. Remington, *The Cradle Will Fall.* New York: Donald I. Fine, 1994.

Chapman, A.H. et al, "Obsessions of Infanticide," *Archives of General Psychiatry* l, 1959: 12-16.

Chira, Susan, "Prayers and Sadness," The New York Times News Service, (re)printed in *The Wichita Eagle,* City Edition, November 5, 1994: 1A.

Davidson, J., and E. Robertson, "A Follow-up Study of Postpartum Illness," *Acta Psychiatr Scand 71* (5), 1985: 451-457.

Desseigne, F. and J. Carrere, "Mothers Who Kill Their Children," (in French) Paris, France: *Annuals of Medical Psychology* 2(1), 1974: 238-248.

Dix, Carol, *The New Mother Syndrome: Coping with Postpartum Stress and Depression.* New York: Doubleday, 1985.

Duke, Patty, and Gloria Hochman, *A Brilliant Madness, Living with Manic-Depressive Illness.* New York: Bantam Books, 1993.

Estés, Clarissa Pinkola, Ph.D., *Women Who Run with the Wolves: Myths and Stories of the Wild Woman Archetype.* New York: Ballantine Books, 1992.

Fieve, Ronald R., *Moodswing.* New York: Bantam Books, in association with William Morrow & Co., Inc., 1975, revised and expanded, 1989.

Gibbs, Nancy, "Death and Deceit," *Time,* November 14, 1994.

Gilman, Charlotte Perkins, *The Yellow Wallpaper.* New York: The Feminist Press at the City University of New York, Afterword by Elaine R. Hedges, 1973, a reprint of the 1899 edition published in Boston by Small Mynard.

Gilman, Charlotte Perkins & Ann J. Lane, *The Living of Charlotte Perkins Gilman: An Autobiography.* University of Wisconsin Press, 1991.

Gold, Mark S., *The Good News About Depression.* New York: Bantam Books, 1987.

Goldman, Erik L., "Breast-feeding Doesn't Nix Psychotropics," *Clinical Psychiatry News,* July 1996: 14.

Goodwin, Frederick & Jamison, Kay Redfield, *Manic-Depressive Illness.* New York: Oxford University Press, 1990.

Green, Tom, "Infant Thrown to Death," *The Wichita Eagle, State Edition,* April 14, 1995: 10A.

Greenberg, Gary, *The Self on the Shelf: Recovery Books and the Good Life.* New York: State University of New York Press, 1994.

Grinspoon, Lester, M.D., ed., "Postpartum Disorders," *The Harvard Mental Health Letter,* Harvard Medical School, Volume 14, No. 3, September 1997: 1-4.

Hamilton, James Alexander, and Patricia Neel Harberger, eds., *Postpartum Psychiatric Illness, A Picture Puzzle.* Philadelphia: University of Pennsylvania Press, 1992.

Hamilton, Edith & Steele Savage, *Mythology: Timeless Tales of Gods and Heroes*. New York and Toronto: A Mentor Book, The New American Library, 1991.

Jamison, Kay Redfield, *An Unquiet Mind: A Memoir of Moods and Madness*. New York: Knopf, 1995.

Koss, M.D., "The Women's Health Agenda: Violence Against Women," *American Psychologist* 45: 374-380.

Lemonick, Michael D., "Cretaceous Parenting," *Time,* November 14, 1994.

Maier-Katkin, Daniel, "Mothers Who Kill," *Miami Herald,* November 20, 1994, Viewpoint, Section M: 1, 6.

"Obsessed: When the Brain Gets Stuck in a Repeating Look," *Chicago Tribune,* Section 6, Woman News, July 16, 1995.

O'Neill, Anne Marie and Leah Eskin, in Racine, WI, and Linda Slater in Little Rock, AR, "Under the Influence," *People,* September 9, 1996: 53-55.

Pinker, Steven, "Why They Kill Their Newborns," *The New York Times Magazine,* November 2, 1997, Section 6: 51-54.

Rensetti, C.SM., "Violence in Lesbian Relationships," from *Battering and Family Therapy: A Feminist Perspective,* Haron, Marsali, M.D., and Michele Harway, M.D., eds. Sage Publications, 1993: 198-199.

Shea, Steven J., Ph.D., Geoffrey R. McKee, Ph.D, Allison M. Foster, Ph.D., and Christopher Bostdorff, Ph.D., *Characteristics of Women Who Kill their Children.* University of South Carolina School of Medicine, Presentation: American Psychological Association (APA), 103rd Annual Convention, New York, August 1995.

Shear, M.K., and O. Mammen, "Anxiety Disorders in Pregnant and Postpartum Women," *Pychopharmacol Bull* 31 (4), 1995: 693-703.

Sherman, Carl, "Prophylaxis May Forestall Postpartum Depression," *Clinical Psychiatry News,* July 1996.

Sichel, Deborah A., L.S. Cohen, J.F. Rosenbaum, and J. Driscoll, "Postpartum Onset of Obsessive-compulsive Disorder," *Psychosomatics* 34 (3), May/June1993: 277-279.

Spitzer, Robert L., Miriam Gibbon, Andrew E. Skodol, Janet B. Williams, and Michael B. First, eds., *Diagnostic and Statistical Manual of Mental Disorders* (DSM-IV), Fourth Edition. Washington, D.C. & London: American Psychiatric Association Press, 1994.

Spitzer, Robert L., Miriam Gibbon, Andrew E. Skodol, Janet B. Williams, and Michael B. First, eds., *DSM-IV Case Book: A Learning Companion to the Diagnostic and Statistical Manual of Mental Disorders,* Fourth Edition. Washington, D.C . & London: American Psychiatric Association Press, 1994.

Stein, D.J., E. Hollander, D. Simeon, L. Cohen, & M. Hwang, "Pregnancy and Obsessive-compulsive Disorder," *American Journal of Psychiatry* 150 (7), July 1993: 1131-1132.

Strouse, T.B., M.P. Szuba, and L.R. Baxter, Jr., "Response to Sleep Deprivation in Three Women with Postpartum Psychosis," *Journal of Clinical Psychiatry* 53, June 1992: 204-206.

Styron, William, *Darkness Visible: A Memoir of Madness.* New York: Random House, 1990.

U.S. Department of Health and Human Services, Administration for Children and Families, *A Nation's Shame: Fatal Child Abuse and Neglect in the United States,* A Report of the U.S. Advisory Board on Child Abuse and Neglect. Washington, D.C.: April 1995.

"The Use of Psychotropic Drugs During Pregnancy and the Puerium: An Interview with Lee. S Cohn, M.D., *Currents in Affective Illness,* Volume XI, No. 9, September 1992.

Van Biema, David, "Parents Who Kill," *Time,* November 14, 1994: 50-51.

Verhovek, Sam Howe, "Dallas Woman Is Sentenced to Death in Murder of Son," *The New York Times,* February 4, 1997.

Vogel, J., "Things Fall Apart," Minneapolis, MN: *City Pages, Puerperal Disorders Contamination, 15* (670), 1993: 8-11.

NOTES

[1] Ronald F. Fieve, M.D., *Moodswing,* revised and expanded, (New York: Bantam, 1989): 16.

[2] Mark Gold, M.D., with Lois B. Morris, *The Good News About Depression: Cures and Treatments in the New Age of Psychiatry* (New York: Bantam Books, 1988): 280.

[3] Jan L. Campbell, "Maternity Blues: A Model for Biological Research," quoting a study by P.M. Nott et. al. (1976), from *Postpartum Psychiatric Illness: A Picture Puzzle,* James Alexander Hamilton and Patricia Neel Harberger, eds., (Philadelphia: University of Pennsylvania Press, 1992): 90.

[4] Tom Green, "Infant Thrown to Death," *The Wichita Eagle, State Edition* (April 14, 1995): 10A.

[5] Clarissa Pinkola Estés, Ph.D., *Women Who Run with the Wolves: Myths and Stories of the Wild Woman Archetype* (New York: Ballantine Books, 1992): 174-181. Reprinted by kind permission of the author, Dr. Estés, and Ballantine Books, a division of Random House, Inc.

[6] Estés, 174-181.

[7] Charlotte Perkins Gilman, *The Yellow Wallpaper* (The Feminist Press, 1973, reprint of the 1899 ed., published by Small, Maynard, Boston): 37-60.

[8] Elaine R. Hedges, "Afterword," in Charlotte Perkins Gilman's *The Yellow Wallpaper* (The Feminist Press, 1973, reprint of the 1899 ed., published by Small, Maynard, Boston): 37-60.

[9] Patty Duke and Gloria Hochman, *A Brilliant Madness: Living with Manic-Depressive Illness* (New York: Bantam Books, 1993): 63.

[10] *Psychiatric Dictionary,* Fifth edition, Leland E. Hinsie, M.D., Robert J. Campbell, M.D. (Oxford Press, 1975).

[11] Frederick K. Goodwin and Kay Redfield Jamison, "Personality and Interpersonal Behavior," Chapter 12, in *Manic-Depressive Illness* (New York: Oxford University Press, 1990): 313-315.

[12] American Psychological Association, *Monitor,* Volume 26, No. 10 (October 1996): 13. Steven J. Shea, Ph.D., presented his research in "Characteristics of Women Who Kill Their Children" by Steven J. Shea, Ph.D., Geoffrey R. McKee, Ph.D., Allison M. Foster, and Christopher Bostdorff (University of South Carolina School of Medicine) at The American Psychological Association (APA) 103rd Annual Convention in New York City, August 1995.

[13] Steven J. Shea, Ph.D., Geoffrey R. McKee, Ph.D., Allison M. Foster, and Christopher Bostdorff, "Characteristics of Women Who Kill Their Children": 1-15.

[14] U.S. Department of Health and Human Services, "A Nation's Shame: Fatal Child Abuse and Neglect in the United States," Executive Summary, A Report of the U.S. Advisory Board on Child Abuse and Neglect (April 1995): xxviii.

[15] M.D. Koss, "The Women's Health Agenda: Violence Against Women," *American Psychologist,* Volume 45: 374-380.

[16] U.S. Department of Health and Human Services, "A Nation's Shame: Fatal Child Abuse and Neglect in the United States," A Report of the U.S. Advisory Board on Child Abuse and Neglect, Administration for Children and Families, (Washington, D.C., April 1995).

[17] U.S. Department of Health and Human Services, "A Nation's Shame: Fatal Child Abuse and Neglect in the United States," A Report of the U.S. Advisory Board on Child Abuse and Neglect, Administration for Children and Families, (Washington, D.C., April 1995).

[18] F. Desseigne and J. Carrere, *Annuals of Medical Psychology 2(1)* (Paris, 1974): 238-248. Translated from the French by Emmanuel Trincal, 1997.

[19] *Diagnostic and Statistical Manual of Mental Disorders* (DSM-IV), Fourth Edition (Washington, D.C. & London: American Psychiatric Association, 1994): 386.

[20] Carol Dix, *The New Mother Syndrome: Coping with Postpartum Stress and Depression* (New York: Doubleday, 1985): 35-36.

[21] James Alexander Hamilton and Patricia Neel Harbinger, eds., *Postpartum Psychiatric Illness: A Picture Puzzle* (Philadelphia: University of Pennsylvania, 1992).

22 Laurence Dean Kruckman, "Rituals and Support: An Anthropological View of Postpartum Depression," Chapter 11 in *Postpartum Psychiatric Illness: A Picture Puzzle*, James Alexander Hamilton and Patricia Neel Harbinger, eds., (Philadelphia: University of Pennsylvania, 1992). In this chapter, Kruckman cites data from B.L.K. Pillsbury, "During the Month: Confinement and Convalescence of Chinese Women After Childbirth," *Social Science Medicine 12* (1978): 11-112.

23 Kruckman, "Rituals and Support: An Anthropological View of Postpartum Depression," Chapter 11 in *Postpartum Psychiatric Illness: A Picture Puzzle.* Kruckman's information is cited from J.V. Kelley, "The Influence of Native Customs on Obstetrics in Nigeria," *Obstetric Gynecology 30* (1967): 608-612.

24 Kruckman, "Rituals and Support: An Anthropological View of Postpartum Depression," Chapter 11 in *Postpartum Psychiatric Illness: A Picture Puzzle.* Kruckman's information is cited from D. Rafael, *The Tender Gift: Breastfeeding* (New York: Schocken Books, 1976).

25 Daniel Maier-Katkin, "Mothers Who Kill," *The Miami Herald* (November 20, 1994), Viewpoint, Section M: 1, 6.

26 Steven Pinker, "Why They Kill Their Newborns," *The New York Times Magazine* (November 2, 1997), Section 6: 52-54.

27 Goodwin and Jamison, Chapter 3: 3.

28 Carl Sherman, "Treat Postpartum Depression Early," *Clinical Psychiatry News*, Volume 24, No. 11 (November 1996): 1, 43.

29 "Postpartum Disorders," *The Harvard Mental Health Letter*, Lester Grinspoon, M.D., ed., Volume 14, No. 3 (Harvard Medical School, September 1997):1-4.

30 Carl Sherman, "Postpartum Depression Has Long-lasting Impact," *Clinical Psychiatry News* (December 1997): 15.

31 From an interview with Deborah A. Sichel, M.D., in *Currents in Affective Illness*, Volume XI, No. 10 (October 1992).

32 Deborah A. Sichel, L.S. Cohen, J.F. Rosenbaum, and J. Driscoll, "Postpartum Onset of Obsessive-compulsive Disorder," *Psychosomatics* 34 (3) (May/June 1993): 277-279.

33 Francis J. Kane, Jr., M.D., "Postpartum Disorders," *Comprehensive Textbook of Psychiatry IV*, Fourth Edition, Harold I. Kaplan, M.D. and Benjamin J. Sadock, M.D., eds. (Baltimore: Williams & Wilkins, 1985): 1238-1242.

34 A.H. Chapman, M. Chapman-Santana, and S.A. Teixeira, "Obsessions of Infanticide and Imminent Psychosis," *Arq Neuropsiquiatr 54* (1) (1996): 127-130.

35 Gold, M.D., with Morris, 282.

36 Toni DeAngelis, "There's New Hope for Women With Postpartum Blues," *Monitor*, 'Practice' Section (American Psychological Association, September 1997): 22-23.

37 Hedges, 49.

38 Y. B. Davenport and M.L. Adland, "Postpartum Psychoses in Female and Male Bipolar Manic-depressive Patients," *American Journal of Orthopsychiatry* 52 (1982): 288-297.

39 E.S. Gershon, D.L. Dunner, L. Sturt, and Frederick K. Goodwin, "Assortative Mating in the Affective Disorders," *Biological Psychiatry* 7 (1973): 63-74.

40 Rose Boccio, "Super Sleuthing," *South Florida Parenting*, (January 1997): 18-21.

41 David Van Biema, "Parents Who Kill," *Time* (November 14, 1994): 50-51.

42 Maier-Katkin, *op.cit.*

43 Sigmund Freud, "Mourning and Melancholia," (1917) in *The Meaning of Despair: Psychoanalytic Contributions to the Understanding of Depression,* W. Gaylin, ed. (New York: Science House, 1968).

44 Goodwin and Jamison, Chapter 12, "Personality and Interpersonal Behavior":301. Cited from the following original source: Karl Abraham, M.D., "Notes on the Psycho-analytical Investigation and Treatment of Manic-depressive Insanity and Allied Conditions," (1991) from *Selected Papers of Karl Abraham, M.D.*, Translated by D. Bryan and A. Strachy (London: Hogarth Press, 1927): 137-156.

45 Henry Stern, "Child-Killer Mother Plans to Rewed: Elizabeth Downs Maps Out Book, Marriage From Prison Cell," Associated Press, reprinted in the *Miami Herald* (March 1989): 4B.

46 David Kidwell, Trish Power, and Amy Driscoll, "Grandmother's Life A Tale of Alcohol, Violence, Death," *Miami Herald* (June 26, 1996): 1A, 6A.

47 Shea, McKee, Foster, and Bostdorff, "Characteristics of Women Who Kill Their Children," (University of South Carolina, School of Medicine) presented at The American Psychological Association (APA) 103rd Annual Convention (New York: August 1995).

48 Amy Alexander, Gail Epstein, and Oscar Musibay, *Miami Herald* (December 11, 1994).

49 "Nearly 5 Babies Killed Weekly, FBI Data Shows," CNN (June 27, 1997), U.S. News story page, html version @ www.cnn.com/

50 Thomas Fields-Mayer, Ron Arias, Cynthia Wang, and Maria Eftimiades, "Dance Macabre," *People* (November 10, 1997): 147-150.

51 Fields-Mayer, Arias, Wang, and Eftimiades, 147-150.

52 Pinker, 52-54.

53 John Lucadamo, "Teen Tells Her Side in Baby's Death," *Chicago Tribune*, Chicagoland Section (April 22, 1993).

54 Jon Hilkevitch, "Woman Gets Probation in Childbirth Drowning," *Chicago Tribune*, Chicagoland Section (July 1, 1993).

55 Todd Zwillich, "Infanticide May Follow Severe Dissociation," *Clinical Psychiatry News* (November 1997): 5.

56 Julie Irwin and Phil Borchmann, "Mother Charged in Baby's Asphyxiation," *Chicago Tribune,* Metro Northwest Section (October 7, 1994).

57 David Hancock, "Mom Beat 2-Year-Old to Death Police Say," *Miami Herald,* Section B (April 5, 1995).

58 Curtis Morgan, "Infant, Troubled Mom: A Recipe for a Tragedy," *Miami Herald* (April 30, 1996): 1A.

59 Susan Chira, "Prayers and Sadness," The New York Times News Service, (re)printed in *The Wichita Eagle,* City Edition (November 5, 1994): 1A.

60 Associated Press, "Mom May Have Intentionally Made Her Two Babies Sick, Prosecutors Say," *Miami Herald,* Local Section (December 5, 1992): 1B.

61 Desseigne and Carrere, 238-248.

62 Sam Howe Verhovek, "Dallas Woman Is Sentenced to Death in Murder of Son," *The New York Times* (February 4, 1997).

63 Gold, M.D., with Morris, 280.

64 Women's Health Column by The American College of Obstetricians and Gynecologists (May 13, 1996). Reprinted with permission.

65 U.S. Department of Health and Human Services, "A Nation's Shame: Fatal Child Abuse and Neglect in the United States," A Report of the U.S. Advisory Board on Child Abuse and Neglect, Administration for Children and Families, (Washington, D.C., April 1995).

66 J. Davidson and E. Robertson, "A Follow-up Study of Postpartum Illness," *Acta Psychiatr Scand* 71(5) (1985): 451-457.

67 "Postpartum Disorders," *The Harvard Mental Health Letter,* Lester Grinspoon, M.D., ed., Volume 14, No. 3 (Harvard Medical School, September 1997):1-4.